The International Behavioural and Social Sciences Library

HEALTH & SOCIETY
In 12 Volumes

I	Industrial Organizations and Health *Edited by Frank Baker, et al.*
II	Six Minutes for the Patient *Edited by Enid Balint and J S Norell*
III	A Study of Doctors *Michael Balint, et al.*
IV	Treatment or Diagnosis *Michael Balint, et al.*
V	Admission to Residential Care *Paul Brearley*
VI	Leaving Residential Care *Paul Brearley*
VII	Culture, Health and Disease *Margaret Read*
VIII	Management in the Social and Safety Services *Edited by W D Reekie and Norman C Hunt*
IX	Contemporary Community *Jacqueline Scherer*
X	Towards Community Mental Health *Edited by John D Sutherland*
XI	An Introduction to Medical Sociology *Edited by David Tuckett*
XII	Open Employment After Mental Illness *Nancy Wansbrough and Philip Cooper*

CONTEMPORARY COMMUNITY

Sociological Illusion or Reality?

JACQUELINE SCHERER

ROUTLEDGE
Taylor & Francis Group

First published in 1972 by
Tavistock Publications Limited

Reprinted in 2001 by
Routledge
2 Park Square, Milton Park, Abingdon, Oxon, OX14 4RN

Transferred to Digital Printing 2007

Routledge is an imprint of the Taylor & Francis Group

British Library Cataloguing in Publication Data
A CIP catalogue record for this book
is available from the British Library

Contemporary Community
ISBN 0-415-26432-4
Health & Society: 12 Volumes
ISBN 0-415-26509-6
The International Behavioural and Social Sciences Library
112 Volumes
ISBN 0-415-25670-4

Contemporary Community

Sociological Illusion or Reality?

JACQUELINE SCHERER

TAVISTOCK PUBLICATIONS

First published in 1972
By Tavistock Publications Limited
2 Park Square, Milton Park, Abingdon, Oxon, OX14 4RN
In 10 on 12pt Times New Roman
By W & J Mackay Limited, Chatham

ISBN 0 422 73780 1

Distributed in the USA by
HARPER & ROW PUBLISHERS, INC
BARNES & NOBLE IMPORT DIVISION

For Ralph
With Love

Contents

Acknowledgements

The author is deeply indebted to many individuals for their assistance in preparing this book. In particular, the comments and interest of Dr Joan Brothers have been invaluable. I am most grateful to Mrs John Haig for her support and criticisms; to Mrs Beryl Williams for her enthusiastic secretarial assistance; and to Mrs Elisabeth Croll and Professor W. R. Niblett of the Department of Higher Education University of London Institute of Education, for their comments. In the early stages of community studies, I received both support and guidance from Professors Fred Burke, Robert Iversen, Irwin Deutscher, and Roy Bryce La Porte of Syracuse University, and generous assistance from Mrs Jeanette Macero and Mrs Akiko Arimoto. Last, but in many ways first, I wish to say thank you to the five people who made all my efforts possible: Ralph, Susan, Judy, Kathie, and Randall Scherer.

Preface

The individual man, since his separate existence is manifested only by ignorance and error, so far as he is anything apart from his fellows, and from what he and they are to be, is only a negation.

Charles Sanders Peirce[1]

The premise of the argument in this book is very simple: men have never lived alone. A basic requirement of existence has been the social bonds that unite each man to others, the most intimate being those of the family and close kin groups. But other, wider, social bonds have ever been needed to link man to more extensive social arrangements. The structures developed from these more public ties have been called 'communities'.

Recently, there has been a great deal of thoughtful discussion about the apparent loss of community, and man's alienation from his fellows. The turbulence of the present era, the speed of technological and social change, and the increase in the pace of living caused by rapid communications and transportation have so altered the world landscape that we stand bewildered and unable to recognize traditional forms of human association. But communities still exist. If they did not, man himself could not survive, and as of this hour, at least, man is surviving. Those communities which are viable, however, are not the same as those we nostalgically envisioned in the world of little villages or even unified neighbourhoods. Just as the complexity of living has altered physical forms, so our social forms have changed, taken new shapes, and developed into very strange and 'unorthodox' patterns. These modern social collectivities are not immediately visible as physical entities, and cannot be readily located, so that we require the assistance of modern social scientific tools to uncover and document what we know must, in fact, exist.

Contemporary community

We shall often speak of 'modern man' in these pages. By this we mean men who live in developed areas of the world: predominantly urban, technologically sophisticated, and rapidly changing. This does not mean that men who live in traditional kinds of civilizations, dominated by the kinds of communities we have known in the past, are no longer of interest. On the contrary, in numbers alone most of humanity still live within the kinds of communities that were to be found one hundred years ago, internationally. But our focus upon modern man is an attempt to examine the concept of community under the most difficult conditions possible. The circumstances of modern societies seem totally inimical to a sense of community, and critics have constantly suggested that community as a social form has been lost or abandoned. In this discussion we shall not assume that these critics are right, but try to establish whether or not communal social forms exist in changed appearance.

Perhaps it would be less confusing if we invented a new word to refer to modern communities. At least we would eliminate the danger of clouding our discussion with irrelevant memories or emotional slogans. But a new word would not assist our search for the modern forms of togetherness. It could only make our purposes more definite, and our task here is the *search*. Our intention is to use the empirical evidence from research to study community in a variety of modern situations: institutions, organizations, groups, cities, and suburban residential areas, to see if, in fact, communities do exist.

A final warning: the word 'community' is emotionally tinged. It is usually equated with a condition of happiness. At its best, community provides meaning and purpose to life – but, at its worst, community can be a source of tyranny and inhumanity. Nor is community a simple concept, a synonym for togetherness and love. Our subject is complex and our search must be wide ranging, for to seek modern communities is at the same time to search for human structures that ultimately can explain man's ability to survive.

1 Why talk about community?

> There is nothing so moving – not even acts of love or hate, as the discovery that one is not alone.
>
> *Robert Ardrey*[1]

Currently the term 'community' has become popular and acceptable again. Although we use the term in many contexts, to refer to an infinite variety of ideas, we always return to the fundamental theme of man together as opposed to man alone. In fact, community may be thought of as the other side of the coin presented in the dominant twentieth-century concern with 'alienated' man. It is the modern fear of nakedness and aloneness that has increasingly led writers, artists, theologians, politicians, and others to seek a positive form of association. Ironically, a century ago intellectuals despaired of the tyranny of communities because they feared the suppression of individuality and personal desires. But today communal man has an attractive image: he is not competitive, selfish, and driven, but is dedicated, committed, and, most important, 'belongs'.

In spite of constant usage, community remains an untidy, confusing, and difficult term. This is no wonder when it has become a cliché and a rallying cry; an analytic concept and a sociological sample; a geographic location and an emotional state. The result is that no one is sure what is meant by such vague phrases as the world community, the academic community, the black community, the church community, or community sentiment. The host of definitions provided more often confuse than clarify.[2]

But in our anxiety to arrive at a definition and to standardize the term by locating an example and illustrating it with specific cases, we may close the door to genuine understanding.[3] Our desire to narrow down terms arises partly because our language is organized around nouns and verbs and we have been trained to think that the unity of the two is essential for a complete thought. Also, if we can finalize our definition, we achieve a type of intellectual relaxation, we have isolated the noun, described it, and provided an illustration so we must 'understand' or 'know' with some finality – and, as proof, we are prepared to answer an examination question!

Yet the kinds of communities that are likely to exist in modern reality are not simple things that can be specified by placing adjectives in front of the term. We require words that combine a noun and verb to refer to a moving, changing, 'doing' thing in process. Instead of closing our definition, we are forced to construct an outline to which we can append ideas or themes. To invent an original analogy to describe this activity is difficult: it is hackneyed to talk about using a skelton upon which we place flesh, or laying a foundation upon which we construct buildings. But understanding modern reality is essentially an outlining task, in which many interspaces are open and system boundaries, divisions, and territories overlap.

Another complication is that the term community has an affective and psychological aura for most of us. To some, this is a strong yearning to return to a pleasant, less complicated past when most people knew community through personal experience. It suggests a personal and human kind of togetherness and is a more comfortable classification than such antiseptic terms as institution and organization. But often thinking about community touches upon hidden feelings of guilt which make us uneasy. We recognize that in our private social world we may not share many activities with others and that we, in fact, contribute little to collectivities. Finally, our speculations about the loss of community may leave us with an emptiness of spirit and a feeling of malaise.

Both confusion and discomfort stem, in part, from an idealization of the concept that has no base in empirical reality; in part, from a desire to find pleasant and positive human forms of association to replace those less satisfying; and in part, from a heavy dosage of sentimental and sloppy thinking, combined with the common habit of oversimplification.

Communities have always existed – and will continue to do so – because man is basically a social creature, unable to live independently. Modern communities, however, are not as visible and as clearly defined as in the past. Such factors as geographical isolation, ethnic differences, common dedication to a total life-scheme, tradition, continuous association, and distinctive life-styles are no longer the sole dominating characteristics of modern association. In our dynamic age, social structures are fluid and vague. As quickly as the social forms are identified and understood, they change. The process of locating the forms of modern community involves a critical investigation of many different kinds of sociability, often far afield from traditional areas of research.

Broadly speaking, the perimeters of our investigation lie in an area of human relationships between the individual and his immediate family, and the vast collections of persons assembled into units identified as organizations, states, or institutions. In this middle range of relationships, larger than the individual and his kin but smaller than the larger wholes of society, one deals with the person as an entity: as a physical, emotional, and spiritual being. The essence of the communal form is a shared association of fellow human beings. Etzioni expresses it thus:

> Man is not unless he is social. What he is depends on his social being, and what he makes of his social being is irrevocably bound to what he makes of himself.[4]

Thus, a discussion of community evokes considerations of identity, of commitment, processes of interaction such as communication and the handling of conflict, and the tensions between the person and the larger whole. To understand community, as well as all social life, we attempt to grasp the relationships between factors – between the concept of community and size, and of place and time. From this study we move on to the exploration of collectivities that exhibit communal qualities.

Where do we begin our search? There are no secret paths. We can look for traditional communities existing in modern situations, and seek ways to fit the small, intimate associations of yesterday into our new situation. We can abolish the old ideas entirely, developing forms of association that have no ties to history and are creatures of and for the technological society. Or we can combine both approaches, using the idea of community past as the inspiration for reform or creation of community present. Incidentally, all these approaches are implied in the work of community development. Here workers seek to strengthen and build strong, satisfying communal structures, using available resources to create and energize human potentialities. However, before we can ever implement new ideas or even maintain old structures, it is essential to clarify our ideas about the reality of existing social structures. For this task, we turn to social science.

THE SOCIOLOGICAL PERSPECTIVE AND COMMUNITY STUDIES: HISTORICAL IMPORTANCE

> The most fundamental and far-reaching of sociology's unit ideas is community.
>
> *Robert Nisbet*[5]

Nisbet's conclusion is based upon an analysis of the sociological tradition, from the classical scholars (Tönnies, Durkheim, Weber) to the modern students of power structures. It is not coincidental that sociology was one of the intellectual responses to the transformation of society brought about by the industrial revolution. Emile Durkheim, for example, saw the transformation of communities as a key element in the revolutionary social changes that were taking place. He explained these changes in social organization by creating a distinction between mechanical and organic solidarity. In the former, men lived in a rural community: persons know each other well, and the rules of behaviour were agreed by and generally acceptable to members. In an organic society, the processes of industrialization and urbanization made the rural community extinct. Men were held together by their differences and their interdependence upon each other. The rules were legal and official and persons no longer accepted uniform customs of behaviour.[6]

This explanation of Durkheim's ideas, though oversimplified, shows their sharp contrast with the thinking of Karl Marx on the effects of industrialization. Marx, also concerned with the societal transformation taking place, felt that man could no longer live in a community, which he equated with the rural, conservative peasant heritage. Alienated from himself, from others, and from work, man could only survive by uniting with other alienated persons to form a massive, powerful class, or proletariat, through which all repressive forms of society could be resisted. The corporate will was to be manifested in the state.[7]

A third sociological giant, Weber, sought new forms of community in the developing bureaucracies of the day. He devoted his efforts to understanding the emerging large-scale organizations embodied in the new industrial associations. Weber recognized that the collectivities developing in industry and government (later in religion and education), could potentially replace geography as the anchor in man's social world.[8]

But even Weberian foresight did not appreciate the scale, pace, and convulsions of modern civilization. It can be argued that each age invents the social form which can best meet its needs.[9] It is possible that, in the nineteen-seventies man is attempting to structure his social relationships (his communities) differently, and thereby satisfy powerful human needs. But it would be dangerous to seize upon community, as have many social critics recently, as the solution to the human difficulties inherent in large-scale organizations, powerful operating systems, and impersonal social collectivities. For we must recognize that community contains in itself elements of conflict, of loss of freedom, and of personal strain. Some modern groups, particularly those in which the term is frequently employed (e.g. churches, schools, and service institutions) may be anachronistic holdovers from an earlier period. For men desperately cling to symbols of togetherness when in fact they share little in common. It is easy to forget how often history provides instances in which community has been used to suppress conflict and prevent change.

The sociological interest in community has documented how all-embracing is the concept, touching upon economics, social arrangements, and politics. The last aspect is historically revealed through the genuine power granted to communities and enhanced at a later stage in political development by the growth of representative government. In the twentieth century many kinds of political power held by communities have been weakened, in spite of constitutional or traditional procedures. Yet those who dislike the centralization of governmental power seek to restrain its growth by preserving local political power, even if their success in this endeavour has been limited to delaying and holding actions.

At present, perhaps the most tenacious pull of the community concept is in its moral implications. To share interests and live together requires agreement on rules, concern for others, and a commitment to the group. The idea of belonging, and being a part of a larger association, is most attractive to the insecure and frightened. It can also be a ferocious web of affiliations that strangles individuality and restricts freedom to the confines of the circle. Churches are the most obvious centres for moral communities, but one finds them wherever group goals are symbolic and behaviour is prescribed by ethical regulations. When people refer to community in this sense, there is often some muddled thinking on the concept. Proponents of the moral collectivity seek the disadvantages of exclusiveness, parochialism, and intolerance and the advantages of 'togetherness'. Rarely can they achieve both, for they seek openness and closure at the same time.

CURRENT SOCIOLOGICAL CONCERNS

> Increasingly, the role of the social scientist will be to assert the *absence* of knowledge on many urgent issues of the turbulent and ambitious society we have created for ourselves.
>
> *Daniel P. Moynihan*[10]

Many people are genuinely bewildered by sociology. Students consistently list their reasons for studying the subject as means of learning 'to help people' or 'to work with others'. On the other hand, sociology and sociologists are blamed for causing student unrest or industrial disturbances. Even the Pope has remarked about the 'unhealthy' influence of sociologists on church difficulties! How can sociology be at the same time so bad and so good?

On the simple level, the response has been that sociology is a theoretical science – the means of knowing and understanding – and this knowledge can be used for good or ill; to maintain and conserve existing social structures or to destroy them. The sociological perspective is one way of examining social phenomena: the method is scientific, empirical, and objective; the data, social.

But on a deeper level, the sociological perspective stimulates the study of complexities: of interrelationships and connections between parts of systems and between systems and structures. It shifts the emphasis from the individual, the personal, and the unit to the whole of society. Thus, when Durkheim spoke of social facts, he meant that there exists a category of realities that cannot be reduced to either psychological or biological factors, but that exist because of social conditions. His example was suicide. At first glance, suicide is one of the most intimate, personal, and individual acts a man could commit. Yet, Durkheim, by a careful examination of statistics, discovered social patterns in suicides that remained consistent regardless of the rate of increase or the year. He found, for example, that people who were widowed or divorced were more likely to commit suicide than the happily married: that Protestants did so more than Catholics: that urban dwellers were more inclined to take their own lives than rural people. He then evolved a provocative sociological theory to explain these social facts – one fundamentally concerned with the nature of modern communities.[11]

Recognizing social facts can have profound implications. For example, when Johnny cannot read at the level of which he is capable, it is possible to study the problem in many ways. If he is not being taught to read correctly, it is relatively easy to use different techniques. If he is not interested in the material, we can prepare some interesting pages. If the cause can be attributed to a personal factor (e.g. health, emotional problems), he can be given individual attention. However, if Johnny cannot read because he is hungry or because his parents are constantly fighting, there is not much we can do in the school, although we can suggest a marriage counsellor or social worker to help at home. But what if a teacher faces a class of forty Johnnys from forty homes affected by poverty? Then we are dealing with social facts that can be dealt with only by social means. As soon as we start thinking along these lines, we are involved in very serious political and economic questions, and we have travelled a long way from our concern with reading techniques.

C. Wright Mills summarized this perspective in his distinction between personal troubles – those having to do with the self – and issues – problems which transcend the person but have to do with the social milieu. An issue is a public matter, whereas a trouble is a private concern. Mills's example is unemployment: one man without a job has a personal problem; one thousand unemployed men constitute a social problem. The sociological imagination tries to link the two:

> Yet men do not usually define the troubles they endure in terms of historical change and of institutional contradiction. The well-being they enjoy they do not usually impute to the big ups and downs of the societies in which they live. Seldom aware of the intricate connection between the patterns of their own lives and the course of world history, ordinary men do not usually know what this connection means for the kinds of men they are becoming.

> They do not possess the quality of mind essential to grasp the interplay of man and society, of biography and history, of self and world.[12]

Current sociological interest and awareness reflect, in part, the fact that men cannot see the solution to critical social issues in personal terms. Rapid social change, mass media, growing nationalism and internationalism, increased interdependence of urban dwellers, are but a few of the factors stimulating this awareness among many intelligent people, as well as within the profession.

The renewed interest in community by sociologists and others is also a response to looking at tomorrow in terms of 'complexity, turmoil, and scarcity'.[13] It reflects the recognition and acceptance of a plurality of groups, goals, and interests, or of what Moynihan considers the 'persistence of ethnicity'.[14] If the differences among men are to be fostered and encouraged, means by which men can live together must be located; and community may be one such means.

PERSONAL INTRODUCTION

> I am a middle-aged American sociologist residing in London.
>
> *Jacqueline Scherer*

Sociology has been attacked because of its 'value-free' stance.[15] Critics argue that sociologists cannot remain completely objective when studying human beings, and that they themselves are subject to bias, regardless of all precautions. This attack on pseudo-objectivity does provide the writer with the opportunity to bring into the open details that have always been present, but not clearly labelled. It is the difference between writing in the third person or the first – what is said is still basically the same but it reads differently.

To disentangle elements of biography from the professional interest in community would be impossible. Yet the facts presented (note how arbitrarily they are chosen: they exclude some significant sociological variables such as income, educational background, religion, sex, marital status) give significant clues regarding my interest in the subject. To be middle-aged means that there are parts of my consciousness that differ from that of others alive today. Born in the 1930s, I cannot recall the more settled world that many people over fifty years of age knew. Even if the reality was not a secure world, and life was as unsettled as ours, many people 'thought' the world secure, and assumed progress would continue steadily and beneficially for all. But at the same time I knew a less sophisticated era than those who are now under twenty-five. Each of us is a creature of historical moments: and the time at which our biography exists profoundly affects the determination of our ideas.

The observation that I am a citizen of the United States is revealing, since American culture is pluralistic, divided, and mobile, and the search for identity and association is acute. The American orientation towards the future has probably led my search into the study of modern communities rather than those of the past.

Finally, to note that I live in cosmopolitan London suggests that I am a stranger in a national community or, sociologically speaking, 'a marginal person', that my ideas are influenced by the place in which I gather information, and that I know personally the questions of mobility, geographical dislocation, and change.

These three pieces of biography illustrate how the effects of private interest, experience, and training develop a bias or an approach to social phenomena, and that attempts to claim pure 'objectivity' are foolhardy. But admitting to a personal stance does not invalidate the search. Some critics of the sociological perspective argue that because the study of man cannot be purely objective, it cannot claim to be scientific, naïvely assuming that science is itself exact, objective, and correct in content and methodology. The value of the sociological perspective is that it raises fundamental questions that need to be examined critically, and not that it provides simple answers to the difficult and challenging issues that face mankind.

Increasingly, modern man has had to rely upon specialists to deal with complex social problems. Specialists, in turn, have access to an incredible amount of new data and materials, spending a good part of their time in reading and studying simply to keep abreast of the developments within their field. All trends suggest that this tendency will increase in intensity in years to come. Unless some specialists, however, take time from studying and learning to explain to non-specialists exactly what they are doing and where they are, it will become impossible to bridge the gulf between the intelligent amateur citizen and the specialist professional.

This book is an attempt at translation. It is written for the person who is interested in community and concerned with the ways in which human associations develop in modern society. As a translation, the discussion tries to simplify diverse themes and has severe limitations. It is particularly difficult to condense the findings of a community study into a few paragraphs without making the example appear superficial. The fault lies not in the research, but in the condensation and simplification. Bearing in mind that all translations present some disadvantages, and that efforts to simplify often distort, I still believe that the need for general explanations of important sociological understandings outranks the charge of trivialization, just as I believe that the need to study the ways in which we can develop new forms of social existence in a complex and turbulent world justifies the exploration of contemporary communities.

FROM ILLUSION TO REALITY: THE SEARCH STRATEGY

It may assist the reader to know how the search for community is organized in the pages ahead. The first steps in exploration were based upon a false lead: namely, that community and geography were related. This encouraged several unwarranted assumptions because community appeared to be similar to the rural village of the past. Elements of that village, such as small population, common culture, natural boundaries isolating the village from other places and different social arrangements, seemed to be a necessary part of the concept. The geographical link also encouraged romanticizing the past, glorifying the small and rejecting the city and the complex society that evolved from the village because they did not provide a safe, personal, and understandable image that could be substituted. More seriously, however, I joined with others who had found in the link between place and community the justification for declaring that community was finished, and writing, prematurely, its death-warrant. False images stifled our imagination and we accepted an outmoded model as the source of research guidelines. We followed the anthropologists, substituting city neighbourhoods for tribal units, or adopting the small-scale study of selected cultural units – distinctive either linguistically, culturally, or religiously – as examples of complex social processes, rather than the complex reality itself. If one explores wearing socially conditioned blinkers and uses techniques developed for simple, isolated contexts, it is no wonder that nothing is found.

Only after I recognized, belatedly to be sure, that geography has taken on new dimensions in technological societies, did it make sense to begin to search for community in contemporary societies. But once again, I took a misleading trail. This time, in my desire to adopt quantifiable factors as a basis for locating community, I sought numerical guidelines based upon size. Only when the reality of quantitative variability and relativity became evident, did I abandon this fascinating, but barren, avenue of exploration.

Then, I nearly made a third error, which would have brought me to the place where many social scientists congregate: the realm of sociological illusion. If we accept that man is totally alienated from other human beings, and that he exists in a state of anomie from which no rescue is possible, the only viable community is one based upon a psychological attitude: a feeling of togetherness and an atmosphere of sharing without an empirical reality in social structure. In this view, community is an intangible quality or by-product of interaction unsuitable for analysis. To avoid this familiar path requires questioning these assumptions and to note that there are human beings who live satisfying, productive lives in forms of social organization that could be termed modern communities. This belief, based partly on faith, but also upon empirical evidence,[16] changed the entire nature of the search. The paths investigated included an examination of the principles of social structure to determine how problems of conflict and power are handled; to the complexities of communal boundaries and of identification of numbers from both within and without. Everywhere, I was fascinated with the merging of social forms into each other; of organizations and institutions; of professional roles and multiple bonding. I entered into the confusion of development by trying to understand the relationship between communities and families.

These chapters are arranged in order of the search, beginning with my own two negative explorations of place and size, and leading by means of case studies through the problems of identification, boundaries, and structure into less familiar areas raised by issues of social bonding, integration of roles, and qualitative selection among messages. I ended the search with an examination of bearings.

This search strategy may be too far-ranging and encompassing to meet the canons of precision demanded by colleagues in sociology, and too diffuse for many readers who view community as the answer to a multitude of problems. Many see community as the means by which issues of loneliness, impersonality, bigness, and loss of power can be redressed. Others use community as the means of dropping out of complexity or as a context within which to find the personal acceptance and recognition denied in other situations. This view of community as THE ANSWER gives any communal effort an impetus, an atmosphere of hope, and a reservoir of interest that will be missing in more objective efforts at sorting out ideas and experiences.

But in another sense, the search strategy is at the heart of the community studies tradition in which community is viewed as an instrument for change. Many frustrated reformers and revolutionaries, who have tried without success to bring about change, see community as a strategy to further these ends. It is thought of as an intermediate stage in social revolution, where embattled warriors rest and restore their strength, experiment, study and gain practical understandings while awaiting events which may push the rest of society towards a social transformation. The fervour of those building new communities must be understood as an attempt to *do something* to meet important social needs.

My search did lead to the recognition that community, in its many forms, remains a model for action. I did not find that contemporary communities provide the answers to many of the problems of living in a technological society, nor did I find communities to be the salvation of frustrated man. But I did find that the development of communal forms begins in the everyday realities of contemporary life, and is useful and important. In sum, my search led from illusion to reality.

2 Community and place

The village, the city, and suburbia

I saw the city and it terrified me. There was something monstrous about it.

John Steinbeck[1]

Men, like trees, need roots. The obvious parallel is that men must find a soil in which to root themselves, and that groups of men living together can create a social attachment to a particular locality. This is historically the fundamental connection between place and community.

This link has been severed by the revolutionary implications of scientific understandings. Two of man's most important concepts – space and time – have been shown to be relative and variable aspects of matter, rather than permanent and stable qualities. Place, once simply a location in space, became not a fixed point, but changeable in accordance with the individual view.

This intellectual insight has been reinforced by technological realities. As man developed the means to move about the globe quickly and to communicate instantly along international networks, he was no longer tied to any one specific place. The more rapidly he travelled, the more often he moved, the less it mattered exactly where he was at the moment. He had reached a stage where he was able to abandon his community of place and substitute newer forms of social organization. These bind him socially while permitting him to be physically free.

The end of place chains gave man a new flexibility, but the fluttering leaf has as many problems as the rooted plant. Man can now choose between alternative types of community. If he prefers a community of interest, he is able to find such by entering into an absorbing profession or joining with others who share his economic interests. If he seeks political or religious bonds to unite him with others, he can adopt these as well. He is also free to build communities of location similar to those which existed in the past. But too often modern man has become so bewildered by choices that he seems more confused than liberated.

Let us pause briefly to consider the nature of modern mobility. The term refers to the ability of man to move about and thereby to experience different environments. But how man moves, or the style of his mobility, is determined by many factors. Social class has a significant effect on mobility patterns and the movements of the poor are not the same as those of the rich. Within a given location, the poor restrict their everyday world to a specific locality usually dominated by peer groups and kin contacts, or workmates and others locally based. In the event of a move to another town or country the poor re-establish themselves in new situations, where once again they are restricted to the locality. Middle-class 'movers', however, have become cosmopolitan, building networks of social relationships in ever wider regions. Different kinds of mobility create different social structures: the affluent build attractive retirement villages, the poor farm-worker migrating to the city creates a slum village in the heart of the urban centre. Some mobility is forced whereas some is brought about by a conscious desire for a change, or a second chance. Paul and Gordon Cullen summarize these 'paradoxes of mobility' by stating that people vary in their need to be mobile, their differing abilities to move, and their desire to be mobile.[2]

Another significant factor in modern man's mobility is psychological mobility, brought about largely through mass communications. Residents may have little desire to leave their hamlet, but they seldom wish to escape from radio and television entertainment. The latter encompasses the world, and in spite of selective perception, which screens out those aspects of viewing experiences which we cannot psychologically accept, the overall impact is generally to prepare us for a different world. As the flight to the moon symbolizes, the future is one of movement and change, and to remain a viable social form, community will be further divorced from place.

There have always been some communities without traditional place ties, such as those of gipsies and desert nomads. Proponents of place like to point out, however, that even the wandering gipsies admit that much of the travelling is caused by the prejudice of local residents, and allowed a choice, they would change only four times within a year. The itinerant gipsy recognizes that by remaining within a known territory he is better able to earn a living.[3] Nomad communities, in fact, represent traditional mobility patterns that are not akin to modern placelessness.

One term that has often been used to describe the kinds of organizations that develop among people when these are not tied to geography has been the word 'communality'.[4] This refers to social nearness regardless of physical distance. Communality is a way of focusing upon other kinds of mobility besides the spatial, such as social mobility within and between classes and cultural mobility within and between particular groups and wider collectivities.[5]

What is the effect of sustained, continuous, massive mobility upon traditional geographical communities? First, mobility makes choice possible: the person can reject one community in favour of another. As a result, modern communities are not the stable, enduring collectivities of the past, rooted to a fixed place, and fixed in both composition and direction. Mobility also makes it possible for modern man to belong to several different types of association at the same time and, possibly, to more than one community. It also means that the factors in life governing man's choices – his life-style, wealth, education, and personality – influence his choice of community, replacing as determinants of membership the traditional items of geography and local culture. The selections which any one person makes during his lifetime reflect man's ability to become totally involved in a community at one time, and less so at others.

Some of our difficulties in conceiving of community distinct from geography arise from past habits of studying little communities using historical and anthropological approaches. Another obstacle has been an unreal image of the small rural community and an exaggerated idea of urban confusion and degradation. It is important, then, to look briefly at both of these common obstacles to understanding.

THE 'GOOD' RURAL IMAGE

> The stereotype of rural life embodies notions of close kinship and friendship ties, of intimate and self-satisfying face to face relationships, of stability, simplicity, honesty, integrity, concern for associates, and other attributes of tightly knit groups.
>
> *Anselm Strauss*

Strauss reached this conclusion after a review of the literary sources of the 'good' rural theme in America. This is a one-sided picture of country life, overlooking other attributes, such as rural suspicion and conservatism, deep prejudice, and significantly, the rural dwellers' lack of freedom to select between alternative ways of living.[6]

The predominance of this view over an opposite approach to urban life was not coincidental. C. Wright Mills noted its existence among American social scientists. Most of the men writing about American society were themselves born in small towns, or on farms near small towns; three-quarters spent their childhood in agricultural states. Their rural bias is best expressed in their discussion of socialization, as Mills notes:

> If he is socialized, the individual thinks of others and is kindly towards them. He does not brood or mope about but is somewhat extrovert, eagerly participating in his community's institutions. His mother and father were not divorced, nor was his home ever broken . . . The less abstract the trades and needs of the 'adjusted man' are, the more they gravitate toward the norms of independent middle class persons usually living out Protestant ideals in the small towns of America.[7]

Furthermore, the small village was a more comfortable home to those persons and groups concerned with maintaining moral restraints upon personal behaviour. City life replaced a personal society in which all persons were known to each other with one that highlighted impersonality and anonymity. These qualities gave the city an air of excitement and danger, but they also provided the resident with a new kind of freedom, for it became impossible to retain checks upon any individual as tightly as had been the case in the close-knit smaller community. One of the many ways in which the village responded to the attractiveness of urban freedom was to develop pictures of city evilness. These simultaneously suggested country purity.[8] Moreover, the integrity and power of the small community image was enhanced by the genuine ugliness and human misery of the early cities. Research suggests that, historically, the rural counterparts of industrial cities were also full of agony, despair, and suffering; however, novelists, painters, religious leaders, and intellectuals who evoked the 'pure' country' theme for over one hundred years often neglected this part of the rural image.[8]

THE CITY

> Paradoxical as it may seem, the city as a type of community may be less important in the modern world than in earlier periods, despite the fact that most societies are becoming increasingly urbanized in a cultural and sociological-psychological sense. The justification for such a proposition comes from the fact that communities – rural and urban alike – are immersed in the institutionalized networks of the larger society and are no longer detached or semi-isolated units related to the outside world only by tenuous connections.
>
> *Noel Gist and Silvia Fava*[9]

Urbanization, according to Greer, is used as a summary term for three different processes: the growth of cities, the increase in scale of society, and the culture of city-dwellers. The last two aspects of urbanization affect all communities, modern and traditional, tied to place or more diffusely structured.[10] But the growth of cities led to a distinctive social structure, measurable in three ways: by the concentration of population, the density of settlement, and the heterogeneity of inhabitants and group life. These three elements gave city-dwellers a new freedom regarding social relations: the ability to select between alternative forms of association. Within the city many different kinds of communities developed – some vaguely defined, some literally at war with others, many temporary and changeable – but since they existed side by side, they could be compared and weighed.

In some instances, neighbourhoods became small communities. Robert Park, the American sociologist who led the 'Chicago School' in the early twentieth century (a group of social scientists particularly interested in the study of urban social life), mapped the ethnic concentrations located in distinctive geographical areas throughout that city. Such units still remain. This fascination with the neighbourhood community led to the growth of youth clubs, settlement houses, and other community welfare groups.[11] The idea persists in ecclesiastical structures by which churches are divided into geographical parishes.

In some instances the neighbourhood does form a community of place, but as mobility increased owing to better communications and transport systems, and to economic pressures for job changes, ethnic groups become mixed and their social boundaries blurred. As a result, the neighbourhood approach to community studies has become less useful in understanding social relationships in metropolitan areas. As one urban planner explains:

> The open society is no longer centered around place based groups: and the very slight acquaintances that do form around an artifical neighborhood are at once trivial: they are not based on genuine desire. Though these pseudo groups may serve certain ancillary purposes (neighbors may look after one another's houses while they are away) there is no possible hope that they could sustain intimate contact.[12]

Nor is modern man's freedom to select between alternatives based upon place. Louis Wirth observed, 'Freedom in the epochs preceeding our own was not primarily or solely a matter of persons but of areas . . . the house, the man, the village.'[13] Modern freedom of choice rests with the individual and is probably best expressed in the form of interest groups.

What this means is that urbanization is still a powerful factor in the scale of modern society and the culture of city-dwellers, but the city *as a place* is no longer the determining factor of many aspects of city life. Freedom, diversity, and excitement have been extended in modern circumstances to many outside of the traditional city – indeed, it has proved incredibly difficult to contain their spread!

GLOBAL COMMUNITY

The anthropologist Margaret Mead argues that community is no less than a global concept of total place. She feels that the erosion of place as a focus of social activities has been so swift that we have been unable to see it in its finality.[14] This is also the message of Marshall McLuhan's 'global village'.[15] He points out that the new media forms provide man with the freedom to accept or reject place as he wishes –

it is not a social 'given'. Recently, ecologists have adopted the planet as an ecological unit, recognizing that many of the serious issues of pollution cannot be contained within localities or even nationalities. Undoubtedly, place limits vary from one person or group to another, and as mobility continues, we will adopt ever wider definitions and boundaries.

PLACE REALITIES

Yet another reason for place/community confusion is the basic fact that people do live somewhere: in houses, apartments, and other physically real shelters. Our fallacy is in confusing personal place – our home – with social organizations. All men require a sense of place to find themselves. Without this, we flounder and become lost. However, this is not the same thing as uniting our social forms to a place. Geography may be the way man has located himself in the universe – but other instruments are more effective in locating himself among men.

It may be logical, but it is certainly not necessary, to conclude that people always try to locate their homes in a community, or to build community where they live. To illustrate the unreality of this assumption, let us look briefly at suburbia: the controversial residential place (and perhaps community) of many modern men.

SUBURBIA: NEW COMMUNITIES OF PLACE

> You do not manage to create a neighbourhood by having people live next door to one another, regardless of class or education. Architects and town planners should not set themselves up as social engineers. There will be many features of English society 100 years from now which are radically different from anything we now expect. But the society will decide for itself how it will develop; architects should follow trends, not try to create them.
>
> *Edmund Leach*[16]

'Life in the Instant Village' heralds an advertisement for a suburban real estate development in Kent, England.[17] Suburbia is a world-wide phenomena, and suburban housing estates have become the residence of many modern urban-rural dwellers. Both critics and defenders of suburbia are anxious to locate community, or lack thereof, in these housing estates. Their investigations provide fascinating evidence of the problem of place orientations in modern society.

Unlike the traditional village, suburbia is a specialized village. Most of the wage-earners work outside the suburban centres, and many are known as 'dormitory towns' or the 'bedrooms' of the city. The long commuter trip is a fairly general characteristic of the working man from suburbia. Other typical characteristics are the predominance of small nuclear families consisting of husband, wife, and children; and the relative scarcity of older persons and single adults. The homes are usually one-family dwellings, with gardens. Critics accuse suburbia of being a social, architectural, and economic homogenization and the ultimate product in mass production.

Even brief reflection, however, indicates that the general characteristics of suburbia may be overstated; there are working-class suburban communities that develop a totally different life-style from that of the upper middle class. Within suburbia there are variations in different groups of persons as well as important exceptions to any average picture presented. As the suburban estates become more established, they evolve differently; the suburban village of fifty years ago is likely to be part of the central city today, and often the rural vision of a country home is transformed into a small urban settlement located in the country. It is dangerous to generalize about most social forms, and the number, size, and rapid growth of suburbs makes such generalizations very risky.

One US building group that has produced more suburban 'instant villages' than any other is Levitt and Sons. At each building site the firm mass-produced relatively inexpensive houses, also providing facilities for many local institutions, including schools, shopping centres, recreation centres, and swimming pools. One of these establishments, Levittown, Pennsylvania, consisted of an entire township; 12,000 new homes divided into a dozen neighbourhoods. Herbert Gans, an American sociologist, studied the development of Levittown, and his conclusions are pertinent to our understanding of place in modern life.[18]

First of all, Gans documented that place to the home-owners meant primarily their houses. They were attracted to Levittown because the houses offered were good value for money. They did not come to find a community, but for three bedrooms and a bath. Neighbours were less important than owning a private garden. In fact, Gans found that

80 per cent of his sample gave the house as the major reason for moving. He concluded:

> Aspirations of residents are usually limited to the house, family life, neighboring and friendship: people have few that concern the larger community and the demands they make on it emerge after they have settled down.[19]

Incidently, in other studies of surburbia, this desire to own a home has been the fundamental reason given when residents were asked the reasons for relocating. Residents of Ash Green, for example, remarked that their house was the best value in the area, or was 'all we could afford'.[20]

One reason that the fundamental privatism of Levittowners was not immediately apparent was that many organizations, clubs, and other social groups appeared instantly. As soon as the builder announced his plans, national groups, (i.e. Scouts, churches, political parties) made arrangements to begin a Levittown branch. It seemed at first glance that the residents were embarking upon a whirl of social activities, but Gans points out that these organizations did more than provide activity. One of the most important functions was to help residents sort out those with whom they shared some mutual interest, as compared with those with whom they simply shared geographical contiguity. In Levittown the population was mixed ethnically, religiously, and, to some extent, by class. (Gans estimated that 75 per cent of the Levittowners could be considered lower middle class, 10 per cent upper middle class, and 15 per cent working class). During the initial settling-in period, residents were satisfied with the immediate neighbourhood contacts on the block or in the street range. But as time went on, they found the need to find people with whom they had more in common, and sought such contacts in organizations. Thus the organizations were not the means of initiating new social forms but, rather, the means of carrying on traditional social patterns. Gans concluded:

> Ultimately, any attempt at significant organizational innovation would probably have floundered because Levittowners came not to build a new community, but to move into a new house in which they could carry on old ways of family life, neighbourhood relations, and civic activity.[21]

A new house, in other words, did not simultaneously bring about a reorientation of the person's social world.

Obvious as Gans's conclusion may appear in print, it is a very profound and important insight that has been often neglected by planners. Many reformers have fervently believed that, by manipulating spatial arrangements and designing new physical forms, they will also bring about social changes. They believe that instant communities can be developed as simply as houses can be built, provided one plans accordingly. Planning has been viewed almost as a sacred process covering and simplifying human complexity. It is true that our physical environment is important and exerts powerful influences upon all our activities. However, we are able to change our habits and patterns in many ways without making fundamental alterations in our belief systems, our basic life-goals, or our values. It is the latter that form the 'stuff' of community, although the former play an important part. Unlike Utopian communities, Levitt's only requirement was a down-payment, and not a commitment to social change.

This distinction is important. When critics complain about the damage that welfare tenants cause to public housing, or profess shock that people reject the modern tower-block flats, they reveal their confusion about behavioural changes and place change. A builder can alter someone's walking habits by the layout of the streets: he seldom eliminates the desire for an automobile. Gans wryly points out that even advertisers have not come up with an effective means of changing aspirations. We might add that neither have educators or ministers.

Planning activities have been most successful in the field of conservation – designing projects to preserve beauty and to prevent the erosion of valuable assets. But most planning has been unable positively to programme changes successfully. William Whyte argues that even in conservation activities, planners have been so fascinated with their own conception of community, particularly one which ties work and home together, that they have not faced one of the major issues of ecology: the preservation of open space. Whyte feels that only by creating high-density, urban-designed centres – the antithesis of many modern planning ideas – can the positive benefits of open space, empty lands, and natural environments be obtained.[22]

However, as Gans suggests, aspirations can be changed by new opportunities. When people can select among alternatives they may aspire to change one for another. Builders can provide opportunities for housing in different settings and to meet different social needs. For example, when footpaths are attractive and available, people may choose to walk rather than drive.

It is the process of selecting and choosing between available alternatives that Gans believes may build community. In the case of Levittown, he found that, as conflicts developed and were resolved, the residents begin to establish the outlines of a community. He suggests that we examine conflicts rather than the common elements of estate-dwellers to see the process in action:

> The process by which this community outcome is achieved are conflict-ridden. A modern community is not like a folk culture, in which congruence between the community and its population is achieved by a widespread consensus about behaviour and values. In Levittown the congruence is much less perfect, and is produced by power struggles which are constantly resolved by compromises so that institutions and organizations can function in an orderly manner.[23]

As conflicts were generated in each of the many Levittown organizations, residents recognized common interests and began to share common aspirations with others. Many residents failed to use such conflicts constructively, and lacked the skill to deal with the problems causing disagreements. The average resident refused to view realistically the inevitability of class conflicts and disagreement over the use of resources, pretending that 'pluralism' – a recognition that there are different life-styles (which need not be threatening) – did not exist. It is because of these shortcomings that Levittowners have not been able to build communities easily, but in this regard, Gans adds, they are no better or worse off than many other American contemporaries.

The community process, in brief, occurred in Levittown as follows. Different kinds of people came to Levittown for houses: some because it was cheaper than the city; some to get land for the children; some to have more privacy than in a flat. The builder provided a house that met these needs at a price they could afford. Once there, residents had social contacts with those immediately close; they then joined various organizations to find people with whom they shared some common interests. In time, those within the organization who agreed on basic issues and values united (a) to gain power over the organization itself and (b) eventually to use the organization as a means of sharing the wider power in the overall place of Levittown. As they did this, some residents found themselves 'in' a community and recognized it as such.

Gans's conclusions are supported by researchers working in housing estates in Britain. Morris and Mogey distinguish between two stages in the social life of an estate. In the first, 'co-residence', people recognized their common interest in housing and banded together to provide amenities required by all. In the second stage, that of 'association or relationships', friction developed, differences of status began to show (aptly described in the magazine article on Ash Green as those who are sniffed at and those who sniff), and conflict began, so that a new equilibrium had to be reached between the elements of conflict and consensus developed from 'a systematic and penetrating external stimulus'.[24]

The important question in the building of estates and in suburbia is the difficult one of whether community can be planned. Some critics argue that it cannot be: community is a by-product that develops when people have an opportunity to interact over a period of time. They claim that as people define their interests and common values or, as Gans suggests, argue over them with people not so inclined, they, develop the critical 'we' feeling that is the first step towards community.

Others say that community can be planned, and it is imperative that we attempt to do so. Only as we engineer synthetic communities by manipulating physical environment to allow for interaction and to stimulate shared common activities, can we begin to establish more rational social forms.

Both points of view are true, as Levittown demonstrates, but both simplify complicated processes. If we accept the community as a by-product of other forces, we must identify what the other forces are. We cannot simply ignore the need for human association, or ignore the possibility that some environments are more conducive to this than are other contexts. At the same time, we will be aware of the superficial planning that has so often resulted from the latter view. Planners have often worked towards a private image of community that was not shared by residents.

The danger of communities based simply on place is that what appears to be a simple link between the two is not simple at all. People themselves are complex creatures, and the social forces they call into being are likewise complex and involved, varied, and changing. For, unlike a plant, man has legs, cars, and planes, instead of roots. Unlike the garden, his development is affected by more than the physical elements of his environment, important as these may be. Technology has literally ploughed up the soil. It is because man's own potential is so varied and changeable that his communities must be more than places: they must first of all, for good or bad, be human.

3 Community and size

How big is big? How small is small?

> The deepest problems of modern life derive from the claim of the individual to preserve the autonomy and individuality of his existence in the face of overwhelming social forces, of historical heritage, of external culture, and of the techniques of life.
>
> *Georg Simmel*

These words introduced Simmel's discussion of *The Metropolis and Mental Life* over half a century ago.[1] If anything his diagnosis of the modern condition is even more relevant today.

We are constantly made aware that ours is a mass society. Material objects are manufactured in *large* quantities; television programmes beam out to audiences composed of millions of independent viewers; huge farms produce massive quantities of food, which are processed into uniform, standardized edibles.[2] Although the adjective 'mass' simply means large or big, unconsciously, when connected with the term society, the image becomes frightening and unattractive. Often we retreat from this unpleasantness by seeking the more comfortable concept of smallness to be found in images of peasant communities.

It is not difficult to understand that large-scale associations and big groups are less appealing to the individual than more manageable, smaller groups. We are afraid of the overwhelming influence, and ultimate power, of others in any association, and prefer to participate in situations where we can exercise some personal control. Yet it would be erroneous to conclude that smallness of scale by itself naturally leads to this desirable state of affairs. Factors such as power are also related to physical size: the child in the family has little power in spite of the smallness of the group because of his weakness, youth, immaturity, and position in the social structure. Size also leads into questions of choice and alternatives, the essence of freedom.

Simmel attempted to analyse the effects of number and size upon human association. He began his analysis of this relationship with a discussion of the fundamental differences between the association of two people – the dyad – and three or more – the triad. In the two-person association, the relationship was intimate, personal, and direct: contact ended with the withdrawal of either party and there was a clear emotional content in the situation. Once a third party joined the group, the association became less direct simply because the third member would become either a mediator or a divider between parties. Simmel then went on to trace the evolution in interpersonal relations within a small group (later termed primary groups). These were characterized by personal face-to-face interaction, whereas the large collectivities were regulated by laws that listed a minimal agreement, or contracts stating specific duties and responsibilities of members. These are features of secondary groups. In the larger groups, Simmel found completely different types of control (superiority and subordination relationships) and new shapes of freedom or coercion, leading to a change of emphasis upon different qualities in social intercourse.[3]

Relating Simmel's concepts to the studies of communities of different size, one sees that certain kinds of human association can take place in the small village that are just not possible in the metropolis. These forms of association have nothing to do with the distinctive personality characteristics of the individual, nor do they have anything to do with the peculiar qualities of a certain place. They are social characteristics resulting from the size of the collective. Thus, in a group of six people, it is possible to know everyone's name and a great deal about each person. When the number is increased to sixty, it becomes more difficult: and almost impossible with 6,000. Yet, in modern life, we live in units of all three sizes – 6, 60, 6,000 – and the elements of community that may or may not be present in each unit remain important problems.

In small units, the characteristics of community can be easily observed, just as they are more observable when fixed in geography. But it does not follow that in the larger areas of human association community is impossible. The relationship of numbers to structure is not so direct and straightforward, because size is usually moderated by many other factors.

These comments may appear too theoretical and abstract to provide practical insights into real communities, but a study of a specific case may illustrate the complexity of relationships between size and community development.

FROM OPENNESS TO CLOSURE: 'GARRISON COMMUNITY'

Charlotte Wolf's critical examination of life in an American military base, *Garrison Community*, adopts 'an integrated system of social life' as the criterion for locating community.[4] In this study, the two critical features of integration were ethnicity (American troops) and the military ethos. These two factors were aggravated by increased numbers. Thus, the Americans who first came to the base in Ankara lived closely with the Turkish residents, and were absorbed by the majority group. The history of the American base was 'one of growing numbers, of expanding facilities, of ever greater self-sufficiency, and of increasing isolation from Turkish life'. Wolf concluded:

> To many Turks that which might have been admirable or at least tolerable on the small scale seemed to be monstrous and threatening on the large. What seemed to be at first a handful of bewildered strangers became an influx of foreign troops, which were perceived by some as posing a menace to Turkish independence and polity.[5]

The military ethos, characterized by such procedures as interchangeability of personnel, restricted community membership during a fixed period of time, an emphasis on status distinctions, and rigid prescriptions for behaviours, became so all-pervasive as the number of Americans increased that there was no escape from the garrison. Social exchanges with Turks living outside the base were few. The compound fever that developed led to serious problems of morale and mental health among the Americans, as well as increased tensions, hostility, and suspicion among the Turks.

It is significant that it was not sheer numbers that led to the development of the American military community, but the fact that the numbers provided 'some of the conditions in which community can form and grow'. In this instance, it made possible the separate organization of people and facilities from the dominant Turkish culture. As the facilities developed the Americans became more isolated, and such isolation was reinforced by the military perspective and ignorance of Turkish culture. The author's conclusions are important in understanding military communities everywhere:

> The problem is not that the US sometimes sends ill-equipped individuals overseas – but, rather, it is the way they are sent. The plethora of difficulties that exist between host nationals and American military people is not alone attributable to individual cross-cultural intolerance and misunderstandings. I believe that the problem is primarily structural, and only secondarily, cultural.[6]

Regardless of nationality, the military ethos encourages group closure. When sufficient numbers of military personnel collect, they are likely to establish a distinctive community isolated from other groups. In this instance, isolation was based upon ethnicity; in some instances it is simply physical isolation clearly offset by walls, barbed wire, and other kinds of fences.

Thus numbers, ethos, and isolation created the garrison. Numbers do provide an impetus for developing communities but they cannot explain the types of structures that result.

This was also the conclusion of Robert Park's reflections upon numbers and the city. Park wrote:

> For sociological purposes, however, we can define the city not by numbers of inhabitants, nor by a given set of ecologicial, geographic or economic factors, but as a way of living, a state of mind, a body of customs and traditions. and of the organized attitudes and sentiments that adhere to these customs and are transmitted with these traditions.[7]

THE END OF COMMUNITY – THE MASS SOCIETY

> *Little Boxes on the hillside,*
> *Little Boxes made of ticky tacky*
> *Little Boxes on the hillside,*
> *Little Boxes all the same.*
>
> *Malvina Reynolds*[8]

Some critics of the twentieth century go further than Simmel and attribute the loss of personal satisfaction in social relationships to the increased size of social aggregates. In fact, much of the interest in community relates directly to the desire to improve the quality of life by developing smaller aggregates.

Contemporary community

An interesting study of a village in upstate New York has illustrated how extreme are the devices adopted by people who wish to avoid recognizing the powerful, large-scale social organizations dominating modern life. Because this study documents clearly the fear inherent in many of the discussions of mass society, and thereby also explains the positive emotional attraction of community, a brief examination is in order.

Springdale: 'Small Town in Mass Society'

Folks in Springdale think this is a good place to live.

Thus speak the residents who think of their small town as a 'friendly place'; 'everyone knows everyone' and all are 'neighbours'. 'Our' town is free from the crime and dangers of the big city: people 'agree' on the important things in life.

This attractive image of the rural village on which residents pride themselves was carefully studied by two researchers, Joseph Bensman and Arthur Vidich.[9] As they dug deeply into the daily routine of Springdale, Benson and Vidich began to realize that this belief in small-town superiority was a screen covering basic feelings of insecurity and inferiority on the part of the inhabitants. In fact, the town was completely controlled by larger forces outside its borders. In politics, religion, economics, education, and almost every other important area of decision-making, Springdalers could not control their own destiny but were reacting to a host of factors controlling their behaviour from 'outside' the town.

The myths Springdalers used to support their local ideology had no foundation in actualities. Not everyone was treated equally in the village as they pretended: several important groups and persons were excluded from the population so effectively that their existence was ignored or assigned to other citizens' unconsciousness. These were the people who live on the 'wrong side of the tracks', the shanty-dwellers. Instead of equal participation, the task of translating power decisions to town language was made by a small group. Three or four political leaders, and a handful of experts in particular professions, obtained and maintained power because they had access 'to sources of decisions in larger institutions'. In other words, the doctor who knew someone in the Department of Health in Albany or Washington was able to reach his contact to gain information, and perhaps plead for

Springdale's interests. In turn, he carried back the official decisions and attempted to modify policies established by others to protect the interests of some of the residents.

The fascinating feature of Springdale life was how residents managed to live with their ideology of small-town superiority and the reality of powerlessness, inequality, and conflict. The authors concluded:

> By techniques of self-avoidance and self-discipline, they strive to avoid facing real issues, which, if recognized, would threaten the total fabric of their personal and social existence. Instead of facing the issues, they make compromises and modify their behavior in some cases, and reaffirm their traditional patterns in other cases. They do this, however, without any overt conscious recognition of the basic problem.[10]

In every instance the researcher's critical examination of the images of Springdale showed that these images were not supported by the realities of daily life. Instead of the quiet town in which there was little strife and contention (or a great deal of common concern), there had been created, in fact, elaborate structures and mechanisms to deal with conflict. True, there has not been a serious 'crime wave' and little impersonality or aloofness existed between many citizens, but this did not mean that there was a large measure of agreement. Whenever differences of opinion threatened to erupt, action was either postponed or delayed for a period until decisions outside the village forced a course of action upon the villagers. If citizens, for example, could not agree on building a new school, threats from the State Education Department eventually made such a building a requirement. When a young minister demanded improved youth services, delays in accepting his proposals eventually led to the abandonment of some programmes, or the watering down of the programmes so as not to offend or, simply, not to accomplish. Given enough talk, almost all issues could be lost or decisions postponed.

Springdale is a case study of people who want to believe that they have learned to exist as a unity in the mass society. The citizens dare not question too sharply the conditions in the town: they resent the intrusion of others, but since they cannot admit that they are not powerful they are helpless to prevent interference. The authors interpreted the psychological demand to glorify smallness, among residents in spite of the reality of large-scale power, as harmful in meeting the problems that they face. By holding to this belief, citizens feel comfortable and reassured: they can deny the existence of the bigness and the pressures of the mass society even as they develop structures and rationalizations to accommodate the reality.

OTHER RESPONSES TO THE MASS SOCIETY

Another dangerous response to bigness is the elitist solution. This is based upon the assumption that, if one is better than the mass and belongs to a small group consisting of people with higher tastes, education, wealth, or other criteria of exclusiveness, one may find protection against the encroaching crowd.

The elitist protest against the mass society may be clearly illustrated in discussions of educational policy. Despite evidence to the contrary, the elitist refuses to believe that more can also mean excellent. He argues that mass education is inferior; that only a few are intellectually capable of absorbing the best ideas; that the minority chosen by such artificial methods as examinations should be the only ones to continue to study.[11] At different times and in different situations variations on this rationale are offered, but in fact, it is one of the oldest themes in history. For example, lower-status groups in society are often the breeding-ground for religious sects: those religious groups that stress other-worldly goals and claim to be religious elites in this life.[12]

However, the elitist response to the mass society is not at heart based upon rational argument but upon emotion, which is the source of strength; logic seldom changes people's fundamental beliefs if these beliefs are emotionally satisfying.

The term mass society itself has become a derogatory phrase that Daniel Bell suggests is a product of change – 'bringing the masses into a society from which they were once excluded'.[13] No one lives on 'the wrong side of the tracks' when everyone is included. It provides an abstraction by which we can generalize about many divergent happenings in a sloganized whole. It is true that man lives in a world of powerful forces that can leave him powerless. But instead of wasting valuable energy by pretending large-scale forces do not exist, as people do in Springdale, or creating artificial elite groups to separate inferiors from superiors, our intellectual effort might well be used to examine social forms that go between the large and the small.

GLORIFYING THE GROUP: OUR ROMANCE WITH 'THE SMALL'

Just as we can locate extreme reactions to fear of the mass society, we can also find instances in which we have tried to substitute small intimate groups for the more public forms of association found in community. The relationship of group to community is that of parts to wholes.[14] Within a community, a primary group is smaller than the communal whole; within a society, communities are smaller than the national or international wholes. In an age of large-scale organization, communities may become ways to break down larger units, and groups may be ways to break down communities. Likewise, in an age of temporary associations divorced from geography, groups may endeavour to become communities and to provide similar functions for members.

When we recognize that size is a relative concept, the implications with regard to community emerge. Most of us know more people than our grandparents could ever have hoped to know; we have travelled more miles and, through radio and television, have been introduced to more people than our ancestors thought existed. Our range of contacts is almost global. Some argue, however, that the quality of our contacts suffers because of the very factors that have made possible this increase in range (mobility, temporary association, constant change). If quality means long-term continuous association, no one can deny this claim. But if the concept of quality includes determinants such as strength of feeling between persons, knowledge of the other personalities, and close emotional bonds, the critics have a much more difficult case to prove. How can one assume that husbands and wives, or parents and children, loved each other more in 1800 than 1970? How do we measure the friendship of neighbours who have lived together for forty years but limit most conversations to the daily weather, or the intense discovery of young students who spend one year together during a critical stage in their formal education? Our own experiences suggest that a friendship formed in a particularly significant situation – when we are ill or need help, or when we are lonely or vulnerable – has greater impact upon our lives than hundreds of daily contacts. To glorify the small group may be as dangerous as it is comfortable. William Whyte notes:

> The group is a tyrant; so also is it a friend, and it is both at once.

> The two qualities cannot easily be separated, for what gives the group power over the man is the same cohesion that gives it warmth. This is the duality that confuses choice. This duality is a very unpleasant fact. Once you acknowledge how close the re-relationship is between conformity and belongingness, between 'good' participation and 'bad' participation – you cannot believe in utopia, now or ever.[15]

DISTINCTIONS BETWEEN GROUPS AND COMMUNITIES

If size or emotional quality cannot be used to distinguish groups from communities, what is a reliable division? Three distinctions can be made. First, groups have no responsibilities outside the unit: group members can agree on any conceivable arrangements so long as they satisfy themselves. This applies to the queue at the bus stop, in which parties agree to wait in line at the kerb or in the shelter; the social clique, or the children who select Tommy to be 'it'. A community however, must tackle the questions of relationships between groups: it must be the moderator between differing parties in case of conflict and, more importantly, the social guarantor of rights and protection for groups. It is the communal agreement in the school or sports ground that resolves the battle between Tom and John as to who will be 'it'; it is the community that decides whether the local timber yard can pollute the river or not; and, on a national level, whether or not arms will be sold to a country at war.

A second distinction is the degree of commonality in a group. This may simply be that one likes to play chess and is willing, therefore, to participate in chess games. But a community requires more than willingness; there is some outward manifestation of commonality – a structure. This structure might be the formal representations of law; it might be unstated rules of behaviour that apply to many different situations; or it might simply be an acceptance of legal authorities who develop the guidelines for implementing the minimum common beliefs. It is impossible to specify how much commonality is essential: communities may range on a continuum from those with low cohesion and agreement to those with more diffuse elements. Traditional communities shared economic, political, and social elements; modern communities may contain only one of these. But the essential distinction is that a community has *structured commonality*. This is the quality which enables a community to become almost more than the sum of its members.

Another factor is that of time. Groups may exist for a brief moment or a single encounter.[16] Communities have a longer life. It is true that some groups may continue as long as some communities and it is also true that communities among modern men may have short life-spans. Nor is it possible to determine how long a community must exist: it might be a year, it might be ten, it might be a month. But the concept of community implies inherently the *intention* of longevity and some permanence, because this is supported in reality by the demands of communal membership upon persons. Since the individual must commit both physical and emotional resources to 'belonging' it is unlikely that he will withdraw without some consideration. Unlike many groups, man's investment in community requires serious involvement and he must consider seriously the effects of withdrawal.

REFERENCE GROUPS

Some equate community with the idea of a reference group: those associates with whom the individual compares himself and who provide him with a social mirror.[17] Teenage gangs, for example, develop styles and values distinctly different from the school, so that the teenager who adopts the gang as a reference group follows gang rules rather than those of the school. Because our motivations play such a critical role in determining behaviour, the importance of reference groups cannot be underestimated. On a wider scale, voluntary communities incorporate many reference groups and, in so doing, become critical contexts for the evaluation, comparison, and support of those smaller units.

CAN GROUPS REPLACE COMMUNITIES?

For several years we have had a 'romance' with the concept of groups. So much of our emotional and psychological energy takes place in the intimate world of primary groups, that we often think there is no need for wider human associations. But it is as difficult to live without a wider public context as it is to live alone. This public arena may not be easily recognized as a community but it is, nevertheless, socially real.

Many observers seek the return of primary groups to the centre of social organizations as the only way to replace the social vacuum that supposedly exists owing to the 'loss' of community. That it is impossible for anything social to exist in a vacuum has escaped notice. But even so, the attempt to substitute groups for communities as the middle agency between smallness and largeness is doomed to failure. This element of nostalgia is found in the writings of Karl Mannheim, leading sociologist Jean Floud to comment:

> The suggestion that the remedy for the anomie of modern society lies in the cultivation and propogation of primary groups, which supposedly act as the nurseries, so to speak, of the higher norms of abstract morality which must govern conduct in the larger society, has gone virtually unchallenged since its prototype was first formulated in Germany in the 1880's.[18]

She points out that it is a social fact that large-scale organizations can maintain a high degree of integration without widespread, intense attachments to a uniform overall value system, and concludes:

> In other words, it is not usually general moral principles that become the subject of doubt and controversy; it is the application of these principles to specific cases. Our understanding of the bonds which hold large-scale societies together is still elementary.[19]

Our fascination with group dynamics has blinded us to the dynamic relationships existing between groups: the frequent exchanges that occur and form the social fabric of a wider association that we shall term 'community'. This is not to suggest that the study of groups has been of little value. On the contrary, the kinds of processes that occur within groups are most relevant to the study of community processes, particularly those dealing with vital community issues of commonality, self-identification, and structure. Recent work on therapeutic groups, T-groups, and sensitivity groups suggests interesting new ways by which 'community spirit' may be established quickly. (In conditions of modern life, the need to develop social relationships with the minimum of delay is vital.)

But substituting groups for community creates the same kinds of confusion as are often found in the 'pronoun' game. Literary and religious writers have often suggested that there is profound meaning in changing social perspectives from 'I' to 'thou', or our social outlook from 'us' to 'we' (The former usually the passive approach to living and the latter representing the active). For example: someone does something to or for *us*, but *we* do something to or for others.[20] But communities deal with the third person – singular and plural; with the second persons; and with the first. In short, we are talking about a social structure that embraces the wider social relationships of both personal and group connections.[21]

SIZE: THE WRONG PATH

The use of size as reflected in numerical aggregates of the mass or the group only confuses the search for community. The social boundaries of community cannot be located simply by measuring the different collectivities that are to be found. Community is not lost in the mass society, nor can the small group replace it. For community represents a particular set of social relationships; public in character yet embracing many private social worlds.

4 Community and identification

Are churches communities?

> All that believed were together and had all things in common; and sold their possessions and goods, and parted them to all men, as every man has need.
>
> *Acts* 4:32–35[1]

Who am I? Who are we? One of contemporary man's preoccupations is seeking the answers to these questions. For in spite of his growing sophistication – or perhaps, because of it – the problems of identification have become critical to many.

One traditional source of personal and group direction in matters of seeking identity has been the church and associated religious institutions. Theology may be considered a sustained effort to answer the questions of man's identity, by reference to a divine being. In the same tradition, religious communities have been attempts to implement religious doctrine through social forms, and churches have developed as social centres in which men use the tools of ritual, ideology, fellowship, and activity to build and maintain solidarity.

DIFFERENCES OF PERCEPTION

The terms 'communion', referring to the sacred representation of collective belief, and 'community' share the same roots: both deal with commonality, joint purposes, and sharing together. Often, by careless inference, it is assumed that the religious community consists only of those sharing communion rites. This relects the problem of using the same word differently. Unlike the sociologist who is trained to examine terms critically before connecting them with empirical data, or the serious theologian who questions the relations between words and church structures, many church leaders carelessly link community and communion directly. But the connection is not that clear, according to theologians Moore and Maguire:

> . . . we must understand that the regular eucharistic celebration made together by people who do not know each other, is only a link in the chain. It is not the celebration of the new community, except in the sense that it affirms the existence of this community and roots it in the crucified and glorious Christ. It is a sign.[2]

Community today is one of the most overworked terms in the Christian vocabulary. This is partly a superficial appeal to the 'good' image of the term, but also a serious attempt to lead religion away from an organizational ethos into a more human form of association. In an earlier age the Church lay at the heart and centre of all life activities. But this is no longer true in the opinion of many. Some have no religious interest, or one that is restricted to Sundays and Sunday School. Many do not recognize the claim of the church to be a spiritual community. Within the churches, however, dedicated leaders and believers remain convinced that theirs is indeed a community. How can we account for these discrepancies? The fact is that a community is perceived differently by different people, Strauss, for example, explained this in terms of a city.

> Perceived the city is not quite an accurate term; conceived would do better. The urban milieu, or any milieu for that matter, is responded to not merely as physical terrain, a bit of geography, but as a symbolic space filled with meaning and people, with significant persons, artifacts and institutions.[3]

SYMBOLIC AGREEMENT

What is perceived from outside may not be the same as members' conception of themselves inside. Regardless of the empirical factors, if a man believes he is a part of a community and belongs (i.e. is accepted by other members), he does. An important sociological understanding is that what a person believes to be true is true to him. Thus, in talking about any community we are dealing with the symbolic images held by persons, and to begin any discussion of church communities, the view from the inside becomes imperative.[4]

This requirement for symbolic self-identification in belonging to a community is sometimes confused with participation. Active participation may assist the member to belong by stimulating acceptance and recognition. But it may also have dysfunctional effects. For example: if a participant is encouraged to join in activities, but feels that his opinions and ideas are not accepted, or that he has not been treated fairly and equally, he develops negative feelings about membership instead of positive ones. To participate without genuine access to power, to speak and know that no one is listening, are examples of a phenomenon termed by Etzioni 'inauthenticity', a characteristic found in many modern social forms aspiring to do one thing and actually doing another.[5] False participation, in his view, occurs when the person is invited to give of himself but his efforts are not accepted, as with the teacher who asks the children to decide about a matter and then does what the official curriculum prescribes.

PERSISTENCE OF THE PARISH

Identifying Community from within

This phenomenon of identifying community from within rather than from external criteria was illustrated in a case study which I completed in an Anglican parish, St John's, in the outer London area. The study was undertaken to find out (a) if there was a church community, and (b), if so, what were its social characteristics.[6]

One of the most serious difficulties in the study of St John's was the confusion about a definition of church community. Many parishioners equated community with the administrative unit of the parish and could not separate out the church as a community from the administrative unit.

Historically, both the parish and the geographical community were one. But those factors which destroyed communities of place – mobile populations, alternative forms of worship available in urban areas, the possibility of substituting other communities in place of religiously organized collectivities – also affected the parish. Today, progressive ecclesiastical administrators have tried to develop more flexible parish structures based upon elements other than geography: by group ministries, by instituting services in private homes, and by developing special programmes for particular groups (e.g. students and industrial workers). However, the tradition of the parish as a community of place dies slowly and it remains the administrative and legal unit of the Roman Catholic and Anglican Churches. Even the substantial body of research findings that document the changing of parish social relationships has been ignored. For example, Joan Brothers studied the changes among young Catholics educated in secular institutions in Liverpool. She noted that when they graduated they were no longer locally orientated and conceived of religion independently of parish structures.[7] Other studies (e.g. Conor Ward's of a Liverpool parish)[8] have shown the difficulties of a parish organization in dealing with social cleavages between parishioners of different social classes. To find the means of dealing with worshippers by using more imaginative and socially valuable social forms has become one of the most urgent needs of modern religious institutions. It must be added, however, that before the external structures can become visible, theologians must clarify the psychological transformation in which man relates to God in new forms of consciousness.[9]

Persistent Place Confusion

Yet even those who accept the divorce from place as a general reality retain habits of thinking indirectly linked with place. For example, at St John's the parish priest discussed the problems caused by a high rate of mobility among residents in the area. He was disturbed because, no matter how he tried, he could not call each parishioner by name. He tackled this task with sincerity and determination, estimating that he spent over one-third of his time visiting parishioners. But in spite of all his efforts, every Sunday there would be two or three people attending service whom he did not recognize. He felt that is someone was not greeted by name in a community, he would feel that he did not belong. In his opinion, a nameless parishioner was one potentially lost to the community.

His concern with names reflects a confusion of many ideas with the traditional community of place from one which the parish originated. He conceived of a community as one in which all are known to each other, where the population remains somewhat static and permanently attached to the church. Unconsciously, the priest was trying to 'fix' the members of his parish. To do this, we usually begin by locating someone socially, or placing him so that he can be identified and our response prepared. Thus the transient population presented a disturbing and difficult problem. In the case of churches, the problems are aggravated by the belief of those inside the community that there should be an almost total commitment to belonging. Churches have always been troubled by strangers: those who, as Simmel observed, are partly within a group and partly outside. The religious wanderer represents a free soul, difficult to hold onto and keep. Since many would like to make churches strongholds of permanence, continuity, and stability, mobility is a particular worry.

Harvey Cox suggests that linked with mobility is the matter of anonymity. He points out that the social demands upon the urban dweller are so high that it is essential for him to protect his privacy.[10]

In yet a third way, however, the priest's obsession with names is revealing. As already noted, many feel that only participation is an intimate primary group can lead to satisfying emotional exchanges, for in such a group each person is recognized and encouraged to participate. However, the satisfactions to be obtained from membership in a community, are more involved. In a church community, for example, members seek religious stimulation and, perhaps, variety: they gain strength and support from the larger collective acceptance of beliefs, identifying with a social form that has a *public* identity. Unlike a small group, the church community cannot be shaped and bent by a few, but it represents an organized, agreed-upon communal view which is more inclusive, stronger, and, to some, more satisfying than other types of intimate association.

With the present concern of religious leaders to redefine the Church and revolutionize its atmosphere, it is important to recall that some people do not wish to belong to such a tight-knit group. Andrew Greeley points out:

> Not everyone wishes to join a new community. The intense intimacy and fellowship of such small religious groups would be too much for some people and would simply not be of interest to those who have decided that religion is not an important part of their life.[11]

The Responses: Members and Non-members

When the church leaders in this study were asked if they regarded St John's as a community, they confidently replied 'yes'. They gave as the basis of their response that all church members had the same values and beliefs; that they worked together in church affairs, and placed the church at the centre of their daily life activities. Some gave instances that showed the genuine concern in and involvement with the welfare of other members. When asked what determined membership, members replied emphatically that the only requirement for belonging was a desire to serve as a dedicated Anglican. Their replies were echoed in subsequent interviews with active members.

However, when nearby residents were questioned about the church as a community, the replies were very different. Most of these residents, nominally Church of England members, did not see the church as a community at all. They saw it as a group or as an organization – or simply as a 'church' but felt that any community group would be more inclusive than St John's. Of all 31 non-members questioned, 29 felt that St John's was not a community; of the 13 leaders (excluding the priest) and 4 members, all felt that St John's *was* a community.

In summary, those members actually participating in and leading church activities felt strongly that they belonged to a community; those less identified with the church were less certain about its communal nature, and those outside or not belonging felt that there was no community at all.

It appeared that one decided whether or not St John's was a community depending upon whether or not one was a member. In simple terms, it was a matter of self-identification: if a person feels he is a member of a community, if others accept him and recognize him as a part of the collective, he belongs; if he does not feel he belongs, no amount of discussion will change his mind. The ultimate test of membership is in the mind of the member.

Membership, Participation, and Scope

At St John's the persistent problem of stimulating more active participation in church activities was solved in an interesting way. The majority of adult members were professional workers with demanding careers, compounded by a significant amount of time spent in travel to London. The church leaders therefore decided to reduce the number of activities and concentrate on only a few. Accordingly, all 'social' activities (meaning sociability) in the church were curtailed. For example, because many members believed that most of the young children between eight and eighteen attended boarding school, they scheduled few youth activities. At the time of the study there were the following sponsored activities: a monthly fellowship meeting for adults, a young-adult service-group meeting which also conducted a Saturday play class for children under eight, weekly play groups in members' homes for very small children, and a 'Helping Hands' service organization which worked in conjunction with other churches to provide transportation and assistance for the old and sick. The intention was to make the activities more effective by reducing the number attempted. One notes, in passing, that these activities are not relevant to many outside the church group, but have their greatest impact within the collective.

The result of restricting the number of activities was, in fact, to reduce the scope of the community. In sociological terms a community with a narrow scope is one in which the lives of members are affected on a limited basis. In contrast, a community with a wide scope in one in which the lives of members are completely dominated by their membership.[12]

Problems of scope are particularly difficult for members of church communities. Those dedicated to religion begin with the assumption that the church is the focus and most important part of life. Those who are dedicated find it difficult to accept those who will not commit themselves fully and who wish to decrease the scope of the community in their daily activities. Religious leaders continually lament the loss of commitment among members and ask believers to give more of themselves to the church. But members often divide their energy, interest, and concern between the church community and other outlets. Within the church, those 'committed' define obligations differently and may prefer to serve outside the traditional religious areas (e.g. non-local, non-denominational – even non-theological).

Where the communal commitment is a voluntary act, it can be withheld. Increasingly, members limit their membership within the church community and thereby come to perceive belonging to the church in the same light as belonging – not to a community – but to an organization in which they perform a minimal number of obligations and services and commit few resources. There is a growing tendency to bypass religious communities completely. Thus the arguments within the community over the degree of commitment (exemplified by Roman Catholic debates over celibacy) are serious and important. Traditionally, religious communities have refused to accept degrees of belonging with ease. Yet the modern community as a realistic social form must exist, no matter how unwillingly, within a social context in which belonging cannot be coerced. Some call this a loss of authority, and others the beginning of freedom.

ST JOHN'S – A VIEW FROM OUTSIDE

The sociologist studying a community must work with all data available. This rightly includes the understandings, beliefs, and comments of the members of a community and the view of the community held by those inside. However, other data must also be used, including field observations, written documents and other records, analysis of policy letters, financial statements, census figures, and other related information.[13] In the study of St John's, the interviews with interested persons were supplemented by the examination of all parish publications for three years, including notices, newsletters, and magazines; attendance at service and parish activities; background readings provided by the Anglican Church, and an examination of some parish records. Based upon these experiences, the following is another view of St John's as a community – from the outside:

St John's may be described as a high Anglican parish – geographically, socially, and theologically. It is located on the top of a hill in the older part of the town, known by residents as the Village. At one time it was considered the most fashionable church in the town, and it still carries impeccable social credentials. It is the Vicar's parish; middle-class homes ring the church itself, but within three miles east and south the neighbourhood has changed to include immigrants, and working-class tenants of bed-sitters and council flats. Although 2,000 people in the parish are nominally Church of England, only two hundred attend services regularly on Sundays. These appear to be prosperous, well-dressed, and evenly distributed by age-groups, with women outnumbering the men.

To the sociologist, the social cement binding the members together appears to be middle-class living styles and values. In spite of individual differences and notable exceptions, an upper-middle-class homogeneity prevails. Although members point out that all are welcome at the church, there is no active programme to encourage people outside the immediate neighbourhood to belong. Church leaders co-operate in town welfare meetings and interdenominational activities, but the only actual church-directed welfare work is in the Helping Hands group and in a link parish where the young people participate in a youth programme once a month. The major activities of the church are maintained by approximately fifty members, who devote considerable time and energy to this work. All activities are open to both men and women; the sermons are directed at an intelligent and sophisticated congregation.

St John's can be interpreted sociologically as a conservative community. When asked how the church would change in the next ten years, the response was overwhelmingly that there would be little or no change. This reply was interesting because the area outside the immediate vicinity was rapidly changing as immigrant numbers grew. When asked, most members did not see the need for *any* change, and found St John's a satisfying community.

In some ways St John's may be thought of as a beseiged community, attacked by the forces of history because it is recognized as a prosperous church established by law and supported by a social elite, and yet pressured by the forces of modernization which includes growing secularism, change, and economic protest. Church leaders attempt to temper the modernist attack by eliminating non-religious activities, cooperating with other Christians within the town and in some service functions, such as Helping Hands, getting to know members by visiting, and preserving the traditional religious values in forms of worship and discussions.

Active members were satisfied with the community and felt that it met their personal needs. Sociologically, this is a restricted community – restricted in scope, restricted in membership to a small middle-class population, and restricted in theological orientations.

IDENTITY PROBLEMS IN RELIGIOUS COMMUNITIES

St John's illustrates in religious terms what is another significant feature of community: when a member is in, he looks out at others. He may see those outside in a different light from that in which they see him – in this instance the member of St John's sees the outsiders simply as non-Anglicans; the outsider in poorer neighbourhoods sees himself outside owing to economic and social class distinctions. The criteria of differentiation vary, and for this reason are very difficult to list when the forms of modern community are in such a state of flux. It is imperative, therefore, to begin identifying community from the inside first. Recognizing the personal and subjective aspects of identification does not deny the empirical social fact of the presence of community. It does, however, help in understanding the differences in perspective between members and non-members. If belonging is a decision willingly given and capable of being withdrawn at any time, it is necessary to understand the many factors that constitute free-will.

The identification of a religious community from within, which stands in stark contrast to the definition of the same phenomenon from outside, is typical of many religious communities. Research in America conducted by J. H. Fichter, on Roman Catholic parishes, suggests that 90 per cent of urban parishioners are not members of a social group but simple of a religious category. Summarizing the evidence, he writes:

> The majority of people do not identify themselves in relation to strangers as members of a certain parish, and others do not recognize them as such. It is only occasionally that the inhabitant of an American town uses his place of residence or the name of his district as a form of identification. Only in rare cases, where a parish of nationality coincides with a certain district can one find a reference to the name of the parish.[14]

He then lists other important evidence to substantiate his observations. For example, there is proof that parishioners cooperate more with non-Catholics of the same cultural level than with parishioners from different social and professional classes, and that parish membership does not provide social solidarity. A minimum of cooperation is necessary among members for the parish to exist. He concludes:

> . . . the concept of the parish community – the parish as a primary group or a large family – is out of date in the American society.[15]

When then do parishes remain? Partly because of inertia and tradition, partly because parishes are understood by those who operate from within – who are themselves in the community. They tend to view religious communities as isolated independent units, whereas the essence of modern urban living is the interdependence and relatedness of people, communities, and beliefs to each other. It is true, as many religious leaders suggest, that by understanding community from outside, observers do not appreciate the importance of faith and other aspects of religious experience, but it is also true that by attempting to study community from within one cannot see how it is affected by the realities of everyday life.

The individual seeks in religion the answers to fundamental questions of identity. Historically, the church, and the religious communities to which men belonged, provided him with reasonable answers. There were few dissonant ideas or conflicting features of life that would lead man to question the answers he was given. But modern man finds many such discontinuities, which lead him to ask questions: he has opportunities to see the outside definitions and compare them with those of the insider.

IDENTITY: MODERN MAN'S PROBLEM

It is natural that men seek to understand themselves by finding a collective answer. Of all the forms of social togetherness, community is the one in which such a social identification is possible. Many think that if they only belong to something or share some kind of social experience with others, they will find themselves. Bruno Bettelheim tells the story of a young student activist who enjoyed participating in demonstrations because he came 'close to others'. He was able to forget many of his individual difficulties. In the course of therapy, however, he described a meeting in which the enthusiasts held hands together. With tears streaming down his face, he cried, 'No one held mine.'[16]

The opposite situation occurs in many educational institutions. Students may enjoy a pseudo-form of belonging: they are told that they are members of an academic community (in the same way church members are told they belong to a religious community), but they are allowed few powers in the running of the university or in changing significant procedures of admissions or examination.

The question of identifying oneself as a member from within and from without is that which Marx described as false consciousness. Marx felt that the only category or social grouping that had reality in industrial societies was that of one's social class. This was determined by the relation of the person to the means of production within the society. In some instances the person in one particular class did not recognize the reality of his belonging there and identified himself in another class, 'falsely'.

The current interest in youth movements has stimulated our interest in the search for identity. Usually the discussion has centred upon personal searches, and the psychological processes that are part of establishing one's personality. But the social structures that stimulate or inhibit the search are paramount to an understanding of community. Communities have historically told people 'who you are, as well as who you are *not*'. The restlessness and determination of modern youth not to accept arbitrary definitions of identity as given means that the influence of communal definitions may also be weakening. Young people may not in fact want a definitive and fixed identity. Keniston suggests that:

> They want to be fluid, psychologically open, flexible, unfinished – they don't want an identity – they don't belong to organisations but to movements. They are highly personal, guilty over hang-ups that prevent love, sexually expressive, inclusive, anti-technical, want participant, anti-academic and non-violent.[17]

However, Erik Erikson has insisted that 'fidelity', the strength of disciplined devotion, is absolutely essential for the development of personal identity. He continues:

> Adolescent development comprises a new set of identification processes, both with significant persons and with ideological forces, which give importance to individual life by relating it to a living community and to ongoing history, and by counterpointing the newly won individual identity with some communal solidarity.[18]

It is no wonder, then, that those in religious communities who cannot evaluate the reality of their existence as defined by others outside – or understand the identity of the community as given by outsiders – may become unable to meet modern man's needs. Just as the tension between person and group provides the creative challenge for communities in terms of commitment, the tension between inside and outside understanding provides the essence of differing perceptions of communal, and ultimately personal, identity.

5 Community and boundaries

The beginning and end of community

Make no mistake, my guest,
Things no longer stand in their old relations.
Ownership has become vague.
When you have learned the new point of balance,
you will be light,
You will sleep peacefully
over gulfs and abysses.

Nikola Sop[1]

As with most modern social systems, it is difficult to determine where community begins and ends – boundaries are generally confused and blurred distinctions located through a social fog of complex interrelations and shifting patterns. Boundary problems are complicated in our search among social forms neither geographically anchored nor characterized by distinctive customs and living styles.

POVERTY – CULTURAL FOUNDATIONS

It is no wonder that a distinctive form of community, popular in literature and drama, as well as in biographies of successful people, is that of the community of the poor. The descriptions of such communities from the inside generally begin with such statements as: 'We didn't have much money, but we stuck together', or 'Times were hard, but we didn't mind because we were all in it alike', or, 'It didn't matter how broke any of us were; we shared good times and bad'. In fact, Brian Jackson, a British sociologist who examines closely the experience of the poor, goes so far as the define working-class communities as 'the shared and repeated experiences of hard times together'.[2] The definition could be applied to many parts of the consciousness of poverty, and is one of the many aspects of social class. The life of the hillbillies, of the poor ethnic groups in big cities, of the rural poor, or the tales of those who lived 'on the wrong side of the tracks' have led to the discussion of a 'culture of poverty'.[3] This refers to the way of life that develops when people have no security, existence is a daily question-mark, and opportunities to change are negligible, The individual's primary life-goal – survival – requires almost all his energy and concern. It is argued that these conditions bring about habits, social patterns, and points of view that would provide both a coherent, overall philosophy and guidelines for behaviour for those who find themselves in the circumstances of constant poverty.

Interest in the life of the poor has been expressed in both dilettante and serious literature, and in programmes of art, music, and drama, as well as in serious efforts at social reform. As a result, mixtures of myth and reality have grown up about communities based upon poverty that combine both valid observations and distorted memory. A critical re-examination of the truth is required, for impressions and emotional memories do not afford sound bases for understanding social bonds in modern life, although they the source of many important literary images.

THE GHETTO

We try to locate the community of the poor via economic walls, believing these are what surround residents and restrain them within the boundaries. Often we also find there are walls based upon prejudice, and lead to the establishment of ghettos from which no economic achievement will liberate those enclosed. Walls are also built to protect those inside against contamination. The masses of China were cut off from the rest of the world for centuries in this way. Similarly, many religious sects keep out the unbelievers, by separation.

Significantly, it can be shown that ghetto 'walls' are built and maintained by those outside to keep certain others within the confinement of area, class, or group. In most modern communities, boundaries are established by the members from *inside* in order to pursue their own interests.

Generally, however, the community of the poor is contained by other visible restraints than physical walls. These develop, as Jackson suggests, from work, the old poverty cycle, neighbourhood, and the extended family to the 'settled structure of community'.[4] This structure is revealed outwardly in different kinds of architectural styles and subtly through variants in the language. The British sociologist, Basil Bernstein, has demonstrated that children in poorer environments tend to develop a restricted linguistic code; that is, these children use short direct statements, with few complicated clause structures, and employ many personal pronouns; whereas middle-class children can use language not only in this way, but also in the more complex ways which are required in literature (i.e. academic) situations. This has emotional as well as academic and intellectual consequences.[5]

THE SLUM

It is usually not necessary to adopt elaborate measures to locate the poor, for their economic disadvantages tend to force poor people to congregate together. In American literature the expression 'slum' defines the residential area of the poor, but the term, in itself, is complex. Poverty, alone, does not make a slum: it is dirt, disease, crime, and loss of hope. Many areas of the world, for example, are more drab and physically run-down than those labeled slums. Even the factor of density cannot be exploited, for the closely packed Japanese do not live in 'slums'. It is characteristically American because it implies a dead end; one has to get out of a slum, move on, linking physical mobility with the American pattern of social mobility. When the Pole is 'Americanized' he buys his own home outside the slum; the white-collar man who has 'made it' gets farther and farther out to suburbia. The fact that present slums, for racial reasons, have become slums from which many cannot move out has finally forced American social thinking to grapple with community issues similar to those concerning British researchers in Bethnal Green or Huddersfield. In more stable, less mobile societies, this has been a fact of social analysis for a much longer period of time.

Irwin Deutscher has illustrated that a slum is a social fact: not an image, a slogan, or a social scientific creation. He points out that in Syracuse, a city in New York state, the 15th ward, a particular geographical location in the city, has been inhabited in the last hundred years by a variety of ethnic groups: Irish, Italian, Poles, now Black Americans. Throughout this century an analysis of police records shows that this section of the City has had the highest crime rate and the most serious health problems. The crime statistics have been consistent, in spite of changes in ethnic make-up, and many physical changes, particularly in housing (a change from single frame homes to multiple houses, apartments, including low-cost public housing facilities). One cannot explain the 15th ward by anything except the understanding of the social conditions affecting residents in that area.[6]

One may start to look for the slum in any city by noting poor housing. It has become increasingly difficult in many Western urban areas to point out poverty in particular individuals by their outward appearance, because mass production has enabled many of the poor to maintain a general look of personal well-being. It requires a second look to see the almost invariable evidences of poverty – poor teeth, malnutrition, or altitudes of despair and helplessness, but they have been documented. One of the biggest problems in the United States has been to convince affluent citizens that poverty does, in fact, exist on a wide scale. Since the average prosperous American has never directly seen someone starving on the streets, or walking about in rags, and can drive by the poorer residential areas in his heated automobile, he finds it difficult to equate the official statistics on the poor with his own personal experience. Mobility has dimmed his vision and restricted his contacts. Similarly, in Britain many citizens are enveloped in a cloak of satisfaction based upon the belief that the welfare state has eliminated poverty, believing that there no longer exists deprivation and severe social inequity. The constant bitter charges by the Child Poverty Action Group are based upon the recognition that the poor have gained little in the last few years.[7]

IMAGES OF POOR COMMUNITIES

Nor are the communities in which the poor collect homogeneous groupings, but they are as varied as the people who come together. Depending upon the predisposition of the observer, the pictures range from the good to the bad. In the 'good' image, the poor community has many social strengths based upon a rich, earthy culture and a social world in which companionship, friendship, and togetherness are abundant. Albeit this culture cannot be judged by middle-class standards, it is pictured as having many valuable assets. The 'poor' tolerate self-expression and emotional release, encouraging man to enjoy the moment while it is there, allowing for an intensity of feelings which would not be acceptable in more repressive atmospheres. In the 'bad' image, the picture emphasized is that of social deprivation, of mean lives stilted by poverty and ignorance – of beatings, dull sex, hungry children, unimaginative entertainments, and boring existences.[8]

Undoubtedly, both images have captured some of the meanings of poverty, and within any community they could both be found. It has always been true that when people are attacked from the outside, they stand closer together. If the wider social situation is hostile and threatening to those without economic power, it is certain that they will withdraw to the inner communal resources to find some meaning and value in life. Thus, the child who learns in school that he is dirty, academically backward, and socially inferior will seek satisfaction in the gang that rejects the school's definition. He drops out of one social context by finding another that is more satisfying and rewarding.

Modern conditions have changed the lives even of the poor in many ways. Some are mobile, if not socially and vertically, at least horizontally from one poor community to another, from one slum neighbourhood to another, or from one country to another. Some remain tied to an area, particularly the elderly. Nor are the poor isolated, for radio and television brings global scenes directly to their eyes. It is true that we interpret scenes differently, but a starving Biafran child can be understood quite clearly in Mobile, Alabama, and Glasgow, Scotland; an advertiser's feast can be just as appetizing when you can buy it as when you can only look! The point is that, although the characteristics of poverty are ever the same, the poor man in an urban slum in 1970 must deal with his existence in different ways from the serf of 1550. And it follows that the forms of collective association that have developed among people sharing such a social situation – their new communities – may be different also. One thing is certain: they will not be clear-cut, simple social forms.[9]

It is interesting, therefore, to look at one famous community of the poor which is often discussed – Harlem, USA. It provides a good illustration of the complexity of social forms and the danger of simple generalization in adopting arbitrary boundaries for locating communities.[10]

HARLEM – COMMUNITY?

Blackness – Homogeneous Image

The word Harlem conjures many different social visions. Overwhelming black in population, the centre of black American culture, a jazz capital, a world familiar with poverty, violence, and deprivation, one of the largest city slums in the US, this collection of black people is known throughout the world. Harlem became a centre for Negro Americans around 1900, when the wealthy who had inhabited the spacious mansions of fashionable Harlem dispersed to more rural areas, made possible by the construction of New York City subways. The population expanded during the first and second world wars. This pattern of settling together, common to almost all immigrant groups in the US made the first growth of Harlem typical rather than unique in the American urban experience.

Heterogeneous Reality

But what was distinctive about Harlem was that for the first time black people who had different background and experiences, came together on the basis of common colour. Alain Locke wrote:

> Here in Manhattan is not merely the largest Negro Community in the world, but the first concentration in history of so many diverse elements of Negro life. It has attracted the African, the West Indian, the Negro American: has brought together the Negro of the North and the Negro of the South; the man from the city and the men from the town and village; the peasant, the student, the business man, the professional man, artist, poet musician, adventurer and worker, preacher and criminal, exploiter and social outcast. Each group has come with its own separate motives and for its own special ends, but their greatest experience has been the finding of one another.[11]

Nor did blackness continue to guarantee a uniformity of social conditions. There are many variations among residents of Harlem today: some have lived there for three generations; some are newly arrived from the farm. Most are citizens of the US, but many are from all over the world. Some are all Negro, others are mixtures of Negro and Puerto Rican, of white and black, as well as Indian and Oriental.

Contemporary community

There are stable, secure families next to insecure, one-parent home situations. Side by side with drug addicts and pushers are ambitious reformers, almost puritanical in behaviour. There is a variation in wealth, with extremes of poverty existing besides some mild affluence. In short, Harlem is as heterogeneous as most American collectivities and, in spite of the validity of many general characteristics, there are still impressive differences between the individuals and groups who combine to make up this unity generally described as Harlem.

In the context of current American society, blackness, however, helps to forge social bonds. Black Power leaders, proud of this racial homogeneity, have been using race to build a stronger sense of community and to establish a place community along traditional ethnic lines. Ironically, their success is also an indication of the racial dilemma in America. To the extent that they succeed, it documents the power of racism in prohibiting the normal heterogeneous social development of black people: that it also often fails to cover the diversity of interests, life-styles, and aspirations of so many citizens indicates the existence of many more significant social ties than that of blackness.

Poverty

Blackness is only one element of the Harlem image: the other is shared with working-class communities and the poor in urban areas everywhere: poverty.

It is very difficult to appreciate the overwhelming influence of poverty if one is not forced, against one's will, to stand up to its pervasive power. Stephen Verney described the technique of a Chicago Urban Training Centre in which all prospective workers are required to take what is called the urban plunge. This means that a candidate leaves the office on Tuesday morning at 10.30 a.m. with six dollars and may not return until 9.00 p.m. on Friday night. Throughout the four days and three nights he must live with the poor and survive on this allowance. According to Verney, the theory behind the plunge is threefold:

> First, it is a shock therapy, forcing middle-class people to see what poverty really is, and what it feels like to be on the receiving end of the church's charity. Secondly, it opens their eyes to see that many of those who are labelled incapable are really quite strong, and during these four days they have the experience of being cared for

> by people whom they always thought of as needing care. Thirdly, when they get back, it is pointed out to them that they have only seen what they are capable of seeing.[12]

Many residents in Harlem have taken the urban plunge for life. To some, the shock is particularly severe because they have come to Harlem from rural centres, and know a different way of life based upon agriculture. They have neither the skills nor the psychological strengths to jump directly into the fast-moving urban industrial scene. Harlem represents a halfway step into that world. As sociologists point out:

> For most lower-status migrants to the city, the working class slum looks like an island of familiarity, in the midst of a completely strange environment. The greater visibility of people who reside there and the greater expressiveness and openness of gestures and words alone create important points of initial similiarity.[13]

The similarity between the urban slum and traditional peasant villages has long been noted. For although the slum or ghetto is located in an urban area, its way of life is in some ways remarkably rural and one can find communities similar to traditional country villages: small, personal, and sentimental. However, there are important differences. We have already noted that the modern poor are not isolated as were the earlier poor peasants. Also, the traditional strengths found in stable, slow-moving societies, such as strong family ties and close church bonds, are often eroded. For example, the black political leader, Adam Clayton Powell, attributes his stable upbringing to the Abyssinian Baptist Church. He writes:

> I am what I am because of the Abyssinian Church, I believe that Harlem is what it is mainly because of the efforts of that institution.[14]

The roots of the many of the Harlem Churches go back into the Southern rural past linking a banished population with a simpler moral authority. There are still pockets within the Harlem population that maintain these ties to religious communities but the strength of many groups appears to be waning. This is not to say that all kinds of religion are disappearing. New religious interpretations, ranging from Father Divine, the second incarnation of Christ, and his followers to Malcolm X and the forceful Black Muslim Movements, are different approaches to black America's search for moral cohesion.

Soul: Harlem's Special Culture

In the desire to find a stable moral authority, black Americans react against a unique historical background. Slavery in America was particularly brutal because it allowed human beings to be legally considered only pieces of property. In Spanish American countries, or under French Catholic influence, no matter how cruel the behaviour of masters, the Church insisted that every slave had an immortal soul. This insistence did little to mitigate the physical inhumanity of slavery, but it did permit one small psychological step in granting to the black human being a measure of dignity. In America, even this small step was not granted. As pieces of property, the sanctity of their marriage meant nothing; children were simply goods; husband and wife were denied any commonness. The heritage of black Americans was a loss of basic humanity. Establishing a moral authority similar to that found in stable communities has become a deep and vital part of the modern black demand for social dignity. Such moral consensus, however, does not need to be based upon the accepted white man's values. Black Americans in Harlem point out that there must be the establishment of a moral community pertinent to the values of black Americans regardless of how the integrated society presents rights and wrongs.

In the search for a moral community, one in which there is consensus, many people in Harlem talk about 'soul'.[15] There is little agreement on the specifics of soul, but it is an abbreviation for a complex of human expressive forms ranging from body movement to art, and best known in the outside world through jazz. Many regard soul as a synthesis of cultural, spiritual, and social ties which provides an important set of symbols to constitute the group's identity.

If soul does provide a group identification, it would be illustrative of the symbolization of community in the developmental process. Jackson suggests that when one moves from the view of the slum as a place to the slum as a process of interaction, one begins to see working-class communities as patterns of working-class 'sociability'. This is brought about through such structures as clubs, symbols, and creeds, but is reinforced through language. He writes:

> Working class language tends to communicate similarities rather than differences in experience: it reinforces feelings of solidarity.

Middle class language tends to define in elaborate ways the individual as against the group.[16]

Yet it would be an error to oversimplify the communication structures required by any participants in a technological civilization. It is not a simple task to find agreement on meanings and values in the midst of an urban dynamo such as New York City, and the sophisticated aspects of daily life in the Harlem context. Perhaps the most flagrant racial prejudice of all is to use soul as the basis of structuring commonality, when, in fact, it is overshadowed by as many differences and distinctions as is any other symbolic representation of different and separate persons who inhabit the same geographical area.

The reality of Harlem is that modern walls are made of glass, not stone, and therefore residents can see out clearly. They may be unable to break out without getting hurt, but they have some knowledge of what is on the other side. This knowledge can interfere with the creation of communal consensus, unless, as black leaders envision, the residents of Harlem can be persuaded to turn their backs to the walls and look within.

Boundary Dilemmas

Harlem suggests how dangerous is the claim that men who are trapped behind walls either of poverty or of colour are automatically living in communities. A man may find himself next to others with whom he shares nothing in common but his race. He may also find himself sharing a common life-style developed from the conditions of poverty. Both factors increase his social bond to others but neither, by itself, can constitute a community. For what is important is whether the individual regards what he shares with others as an important part of life. He may choose to build his community on factors unrelated to the least common denominator of race or poverty. If we define the borders of Harlem by the criteria of race we are guilty of gross oversimplification. Any black community in Harlem is not characterized by colour alone. To determine its existence, we would be wiser to begin with the recognition by members rather than locating its boundaries by skin colour. James Baldwin says this very bluntly:

What white people have to do, is to try to find out in their own hearts why it was necessary to have a nigger in the first place, because I'm a man, but if you think I'm a nigger, it means you need it. Why?[17]

Boundaries in modern social systems are too complicated and fluid to be located without an understanding of internal identifications and when we overlook these, we are engaged in simple labelling.

Likewise, poverty is much too complicated a phenomenon to serve as the basis of communal divisions. The ferment and activity currently invested in the branch of social work termed 'community organization' is an indication of the ways in which outmoded concepts of poverty have been challenged. The old approaches of the individual caseworker or the neighbourhood house have simply not been adequate to deal with the complexities of individual, group, organizational, local, ethnic, and economic inter-relationships that compose communal structure. Questions of identity, commitment, and power are now gradually recognized as the significant parts of the communal matrix. To function effectively, agencies, individuals, and policies must learn ways of operating within existing communal structures.[18] In short, poverty boundaries are not painted lines that enclose a community. Rather, poverty is a thread woven into the fabric of human life, worn differently, by some stitched finely or boldly, openly or covertly. The analogy is practical: Just as clothes do not literally make the man, but do exert powerful influences over his development, so poverty defines collectivities in many subtle ways. Yet a man is more than his clothes! Community is more than a common life-style based upon poverty.

FURTHER REFLECTIONS ON COMMUNITY BOUNDARIES

Traditionally, boundaries have enabled members of a community to look out at others from within the social enclave. They have enabled others to know the extent of such social collectivities. The physical expressions of boundaries, walls, have kept some in and some out and allowed a kind of permanence or boundary maintenance. But modern society is characterized by connectedness and the interrelatedness of social forms. Walls can be maintained only at great cost and, even then, not very effectively. Stated sociologically:

Communities are defined in terms of the solidarity shared by their

> members which forms the basis of their mutual orientation to social action.[19]

This is more than simply finding yourself in a common situation with others who react to the situation in the same way. It is only when this feeling leads to a 'mutual orientation' of behaviour to each other than relationships become communal.

Why, in fact, do we require communal boundaries? Like definitions, identifications, and locations, a boundary is a manmade device for grasping reality. When we can see the beginning and end of matters we feel that we understand and control our universe. Modern social reality, however, is not so easily bounded and communities do not easily rest behind either place lines or class and ethnic group boundaries. Perhaps we will have to adopt the practice of some public administrators who try to find ways of ignoring fixed administrative unit lines in order to accomplish specific goals. The problems of sewage, water, air pollution, road-building, and other twentieth-century headaches are not restricted by town or city lines. To resolve such problems *ad hoc* units are often established, designed to accomplish particular ends and operate on a regional basis – in short, the boundaries are defined by need. Likewise, it is reasonable to assume that modern communities develop on an *ad hoc* basis according to the needs of members.

Vague boundaries also suggest that there are degrees of intensity within the confines of the included part. This leads us to conclude that some are more included in community than others: and that some are moving in and out of the boundaries continually. This makes social scientific research more difficult, but it also means that boundaries will be based upon human desires, goals, and purposes – not walls.

6 Community and structure, conflict, and power

The political aspects

> The study of politics is the study of influence and the influential – *Who gets what, when, how.*
>
> *Harold D. Lasswell*[1]

By the political aspects of community, we refer to three important ideas; structure, conflict, and power. Each idea leads directly to consideration of the others and all three are interrelated, but to simplify our discussion, we will try to isolate each idea before combining them.

In discussing these three political essentials in the concept of community, we move away from Utopian visions. For it is only in a Utopia that man could exist without conflict and stress, and the failure of so many Utopian experiments in community may be found in the reluctance to face the reality of the political nature of all communal forms.

STRUCTURE

> We are all living together, travelling further, meeting more people. We do not move along parallel lines like trams but continue to criss-cross each other's tracks like taxis. We tread on each other to reach the same dung like puppies. We coagulate in clusters like nests of bees. And we are not free-falling through space but obey, whether we like it or not, the universal pull of social gravity, the tidal currents of communal conformity, towards the same places, the same jobs, the same entertainments, the same wives, the same routines.
>
> *A. O'Brien*[2]

As this quotation illustrates, community is more than sentiment. Although there is a vital emotional and psychological investment in the maintenance of community, there is the requirement for the additional sociological characteristic of structure.

When we speak of physical structures it is clear that we refer to the visible supports that contain and hold together buildings and other fabrications. But a social structure is more abstract only because one cannot immediately identify how it contains and holds people together. It is a fundamental sociological truism that people do not live in total confusion but create structures to facilitate interaction, whether they are recognized or unnoticed.

Some parts of the social structure of a collective are obvious: a law, for example, is a formal statement of some of the group sentiment. But the promulgated laws and formal representation of rules are only the surface manifestations of structure and one can obtain more understanding of structure by examining other facets of social life. For example, the study of language suggests many of the common values and understandings of the groups expressing themselves; the manner in which routine activities are followed provides many instances of understood and shared beliefs. To understand the shared values within community we must look closely at the trivia and minute detail of what a man takes for granted, for these do lead us to the unspoken assumptions that determine much of human behaviour.

As we begin to appreciate the manifestations of structure in many areas of culture, it becomes clear that often members of a community are unaware of the elements of structure within which they meet. At first glance, for example, the so-called 'hippy' communities appear to be lawless, free from group regulations and restrictions. But careful observations of many communities reveals how members adhere to a rigid social structure that includes agreement on personal details (dress, overall appearance), the sharing of property, accepting newcomers into the group, sometimes a distinctive style of speech or collection of beliefs towards the rest of society. They are not far from the traditional religious communities which have a detailed, formalized, acknowledged social structure.

In fact, the religious traditional style and that of the hippies provide dramatic illustration of the rift between the new and old social forms.[3] The two blend together in the development of many new religious experiments that are established in reaction against the legalism and formalism of churches. However, as Greeley notes:

> Frequently, especially in amateur theologizing and sociologizing about the Church, one would gain the impression that the Church as a community is somehow opposed to the Church as a structure (or institution), as though the ideal would be to have a Christian community without structure. It rarely occurs to such commentators that a community without structure is a non-existent community because all human groups, even the most simple, quickly evolve established patterns of behaviour and agreed-upon norms to regulate these patterns of behaviour. In other words, even the most elementary community has structure and laws. Those who wish to eliminate laws and organization in the Church, and replace them with affection and love, show little understanding of man or of society.[4]

Social structure is an essential of group life, no matter how well covered the details of the structure remain. Because most modern communities have an informal, non-legalistic ethic, we think that it is absent. Add to this the loss of geographical concentration, and it might seem that structure is missing. The example that follows, however, reveals that structure is 'alive and well' even if hidden.

Chelsea – A Student Community

> Personally, I regard the freedom of flat life highly and would not live otherwise.
>
> *A Chelsea student*[5]

British students today tend increasingly to seek the independence of living away from the traditional residential halls. Some educators fear that such arrangements may lead to social chaos and hinder studying, claiming that student careers will become more fragmented and less stimulating if the trend continues. To investigate the effects of accommodation upon student development, I studied intensively a group of students at Chelsea College of Technology living in flats independent of the College. In the process, a great deal of information was collected regarding the social arrangements and communal structure of flat-living.

Perhaps no island tribe has more elaborate social rules and regulations than students living together. Rules range from a written bookkeeping system for recording financial agreements to unstated assumptions regarding territorial rights when visitors arrive. The students have an uncertain consensus regarding acceptable behaviour over a wide range of conditions.

For example, a student who visits other flats frequently and eats meals without contributing to the cost is regarded as the most undesirable of social beings. To a lesser degree, the student who does not perform his share of cooking, washing-up, or marketing, is not well thought of either. Often these activities become specialized functions, so that the student who finishes early on a particular day will shop, another becomes the best cook, and so on. The ethical code that deals with common problems – eg. one must never move out of a flat in the middle of a term leaving the remaining members to pay the rent – is well understood by the participants even if it is not written down. Other parts of this code include the abandonment of flatmates, obtaining new members in the group, the entertaining of company, and financial terms.

Agreements are established regarding everyday details of living. These range from when to play the television to how late on a Saturday members can stay in bed. In one flat, for example, nine students – five male and four female – live in two bedrooms, reception room, kitchen, and bathroom. In order to make the situation tolerable, each student has a particular night for the bath, and special space for clothes and private food provisions.

There is a great ritual and organization concerning food. Students enjoy the flexibility of cooking for themselves and scheduling meals at convenient personal times, although some of the girls particularly resent the time taken in this activity. Money is usually placed in the 'kitty' for breakfast and dinner; or, in some instances, simply for breakfast and weekend meals.

Students who deviate from the flat norms are generally talked to and 'chewed-out' by other members. In two flats, however, there was an elaborate sanction method based upon points which determined the punishment and the type of disapproved behaviour. In these two instances, the largest number of demerits was awarded for eating more of one's share of the kitty. If warnings go unheeded, there is generally a reorganization of routine, so that fewer meals are eaten in the flat, or students switch partners or turn the kitchen into a study area, etc. If the condition deteriorates further, the entire flat arrangements might collapse, in which case they all separate. However, since many sign leases or pay their rent in advance, it is a serious problem if someone has become so incompatible that the group must break up. Often other members of the flat look around for students living together in other situations for the swapping of difficult partners.

Money is a constant problem since many students are managing their finances for the first time. On a particular cold Sunday during the study, almost every student who reported his activities made a notation about what steps he and his flatmates undertook to keep warm. This ranged from staying in bed most of the day (reported by 7) to going to the pub as soon as it opened, or visiting someone with heat. Poor financial managers did literally do without meals when their grant funds ran low, and those students who smoked and drank to any extent found that they could not meet all their expenses each week.

But greatest advantage of living in a flat proclaimed by students is their 'freedom'. When asked to specify freedom, students generally noted entertaining friends and eating at all hours; 'doing what you want' and no restrictions. Often such freedom is symbolic: two boys who stressed the virtue of entertaining admitted that they lived so far away from the college that they have had friends to stay only twice in five months. Nor does entertaining always mean someone of the opposite sex. Because London is an attraction for all kinds of people, students and non-students, the Chelsea students often 'put up' many visitors. In return, on some weekends Chelsea students trek out to many of the newer universities all over England. Slightly less than half (21) visited another college during the two-week period.

The symbolic meaning of residence is one that cannot be ignored. To live away from home is seen as independence.[6] Halls are only a partial break since meals are still provided, there is some supervision of activities, and the other details of living are overseen. But to live in a flat is viewed as part of growing up and being mature – a condition highly prized by many students. In their comments students refer to the way in which living in a flat has helped them to become independent and to stand on their own feet. In many instances, it is the first time they have had to cope with money, managing business details, providing meals and related tasks. They value this experience highly.

Ironically, the students seem unaware of the social structures which they have evolved in living together. When the researcher inquired about rules and regulations, almost all the respondents pointed out that there were none. They felt that they could genuinely do what they wished, and that any rules would be an impediment to communal life. Since they were, in fact, governed by few external rules, they did not feel contained by many rigid internal regulations which had been developed almost unconsciously.

CONFLICT

> A certain amount of discord, inner divergence and controversy, is organically tied up with the very elements that ultimately hold the group together . . . oppression usually increases if it is suffered calmly and without protest, but also because opposition gives us inner satisfaction, distraction, relief. . . .
>
> *Georg Simmel*[7]

Social structures provide means for the expression of another critical element in all human interaction: conflict. Those who see community as an emotional bond of togetherness usually paint their image in glowing colours of warmth and affection, dimming out, as far as possible, the strains, tensions, and inevitable clash of interests that are normally present in hues just as strong. This is because most of us have been reluctant to understand the complexity of conflict and the important part it plays in human affairs.

Three sociological propositions regarding conflict must be noted:

1. Conflict is necessary. Just as it becomes essential for the maturing personality to assert his individuality, establish identity, and learn to be in control of his own personal emotions and skills, so the community must also go through this process. Wherever the person has a choice, when he seeks his own private interests instead of those generally pursued by others, conflict is inevitable. Freud's significant insights into the irrational and emotional foundations of many human dilemmas also brought attention to the many devious and subtle ways in which man is able to cope with his tensions. Whether by repression or sublimation or disguise, man somehow learns how to control and channel these difficulties or face the consequences in mental and physical ill health. Likewise, anthropologists have illustrated the ways in which different types of societies have been able to devise social means to relieve the tensions and problems that inevitably develop among groups. The forms are incredibly varied, ranging from rhythmic dancing in mock battles, athletic games, name-calling, to beatings. Modern man has repeatedly turned to warfare, murder, and violent destruction in his attempts to face the inevitable disagreements among persons. As Keniston has pointed out, many of the problems of poverty and sex found in the Victorian era have been replaced in ours with problems of violence and aggression.[8]

2. There are many types of conflict. Nor does conflict, *per se,* necessarily involve only harmful and negative influences. The range of conflicts extends from mild disagreement to open killing and war. There are long-sustained disagreements, brief flare-ups, competitions, struggles. It is imperative to examine the type of conflict involved and analyse the nature of each form to understand its possible function in any given situation.

3. Conflict, can be beneficial. It affords definite social advantages in some circumstances. Most of the important gains in civilization have been brought about through the irritant of conflict, introducing new goals to the system or transforming it by revolution. Simmel suggested that conflict can build community against the common enemy;[9] and Coser suggests that it is essential to drain off hostile sentiments. Close relationships require some conflict to ensure stability. Groups built on rigid structures frequently search for enemies to maintain unity and internal cohesion, just as they seek a dissenter when threatened from without to maintain inner unity. But conflict may also enable parties to reassess each other's strength and can serve as a balancing mechanism to consolidate groups. Finally, struggle may bring together unrelated persons in a coalition.

However, Coser concludes that 'not every type of conflict can subserve functions for all groups'. He writes:

> The intensity of a conflict which threatens to 'tear apart', which attacks the consensual basis of a social system, is related to the rigidity of the structure. What threatens the equilibrium of such a structure is not conflict as such, but the rigidity itself which permits hostilities to accumulate and to be channelled along one major line of cleavage once they they break out in conflict.[10]

In the words of James Coleman, 'community disagreements are also a measure of community life. If communities held only the physical things of existence for their members, there would be no disagreement'.[11] In an interesting analysis of conflict, Coleman discusses the influence of different elements in community controversy: the kind of event that triggers controversy (whether internal or external and whether it affects many members personally and directly); the content of the issue; and the response that is given to the event. He then goes into the dynamics of controversy, i.e. how issues change from specific disagreements to more general ones and into new issues, and the changes in social relations among members in the dispute.

One of the serious dilemmas in approaching modern community studies is the effect of voluntarism upon controversy. If members are able to withdraw from the community freely, they have less incentive to stay and fight within the group. One could argue that one of the most important modern twentieth-century structures for handling community controversy is withdrawal. But in many instances members are not content to withdraw and in these cases the community must find the means to handle controversy.

Therefore an important understanding among members of any community concerns how conflict is handled. The first step must be the recognition of the fact that conflict situations do, in fact, exist. Often some community members are so concerned about projecting the image of togetherness and unity that they suppress, even to themselves, the realities of social interaction. An example of this is described below.

The Mythical Academic Community

> A university is a community, but it is a community of a special kind – a community devoted to inquiry. It exists so that its members may inquire into truths of all sorts. Its presence marks our commitment to the idea that somewhere in society there must be an organisation in which anything can be studied or questioned – not merely safe and established things, but the most troublesome questions of politics and war, of sex and morals, of property and national loyalty. It is governed by the idea of academic freedom, applicable both to faculty and students.
>
> *Richard Hofstadter*[12]

There is an academic fairytale which has long been circulated about a community of scholars who live together in a university and try to discover truth. Each year young men and women also come to the university to learn the truth which the scholars have found. They live together in harmony, studying world problems, discussing philosophical issues, and stimulating each other's intellectual growth. All members of the community contribute to making communal rule and to establishing procedures to govern everyday activities. This intimate dedicated community is set apart from the rest of society. Members share common values and beliefs.

Any similarity between the academic paradise described and the realities of most educational arrangements must surely be coincidental! Historically, no such community ever existed. It is true that some situations approximate the ideal more closely than others. For example, Logan Wilson suggests that the Center for Advanced Studies in the Behavioral Sciences at Palo Alto, California, is close to this ideal. Scholars meet as fellows engaged in intellectual explorations. There are no departments or divisions; they do not have to teach; nor do they account to any outsiders for their work. Their family status is usually not demanding, because moving to California is only a temporary relocation.[13]

But in the usual academic arrangements conditions differ. There is, first of all, what Logan suggests is the 'normal level of griping'. In universities faculty members are discontented with salaries, promotion opportunities, heavy schedules, the lack of secretarial assistance or of laboratory or other research facilities, administrative policies, and a host of other factors that affect them in the performance of their role. Students despair because of the pressures of academic assignments, dull courses or difficult learning experience, faculty remoteness, the division of subjects, boredom or too many extra activities, financial concerns, personal worries ranging from sexual matters to feelings of inferiority. One could continue the list, suggesting reasons for unrest among almost all participants in the college and university setting. In most instances, the background of unease remains dormant. However, whenever a catalyst, in the form of an event, a person, or even a pervading trend, shatters the atmosphere and affects directly one of these general areas, there is bound to be tension, conflict, and a clash of interests. Resolving the conflict in some ways can trigger processes leading towards an enriched community; if ignored, issues of conflict become issues of combat.

Different interpretations of reality are inherent in most conflict situations. Clark Kerr, for example, labelled opponents of large-scale universities as Utopian. He wrote:

> . . . the cry for community, the cry for integration of thought and action, are cries that call backward to a smaller, simpler world . . . The longing for community, for this fantasy, this pie-in-the-sky, can actually impede efforts to make better that which must be.[14]

Kerr's *must*, according to critics, assumes that man must change to fit into a technological society and not vice versa. They argue that the university must become a community if it is to remain a significant institution in modern society.

Regardless of the specific reasons for conflict (and they are abundant in the structure of the university in questions of teaching or research priority, graduate or undergraduate programmes, etc.), there are features of community that, in themselves, assure that conflict is inevitable: the tension between person and collectivity, between one community and another, and between the personal development of the member and communal advantage in terms of commitment, personal integration, and emotional expression. Any confusion in regard to participation, as in the case of the university debates over priority and status, threatens the stability of the communal enterprise. The divisions into specialities and the introduction of liaison personnel tends to reduce commonality. These tensions become particularly sharp in a situation in which originality, independence, and autonomy are highly valued.

Yet the very term 'academic community' has a usefulness because of its ambiguity. It provides an umbrella under which many diverse interests, skills, and goals may be brought together, so that commitment is encouraged. The problem is not in the use of ambiguity to further ends, but in refusing to acknowledge that it exists.

Maintaining the myth of an academic community has had serious consequences upon educational development. In some cases, the pressures for consensus has forced out debate and discussion. Insistence upon the communal goal over personal development has often led to a lack of emphasis upon excellence, creativity, and serious intellectualism. For every student who blossoms in an intimate restricted social setting, another may become bored or restless. Some students might thrive intellectually if they could conceive of the instructor as an antagonist or challenger. The demand of students for some share in the governance of universities may in fact lead to more communal structures than existed prior to this conflict and close this option.

But the most serious danger of the academic community myth is that it often masks an 'inauthentic' structure. Etzioni suggests that inauthenticity develops from the 'strains resulting from the split between the appearance of community and the underlying bureaucratic reality'.[15]

> Inauthenticity enters when actors pretend that they are goal-orientated while actually they are instrumental, when they pretend that they seek friendship while actually they seek utilization (such as the quasi-friendship of the salesman or the status-seeker). The falsification of friendship or community may be deliberate (as in advertising) or unwittingly built into the relationship (as in the status competition in some suburbs).

The irony of the mythical academic community is that it depends upon a misunderstanding about the reality of human communities. The myth is based upon the belief that within a community harmony and unity are all-pervasive. In actual fact, no viable community can exist without conflict.

POWER

> Power has an inherent scarcity value.
>
> *R. Schermerhorn*[16]

Within collective social forms, particularly communities, man attempts to achieve some control over and stability within his environment by the strength of collective action. Man alone is weak; men together have power. In any collection of persons, there must be an ultimate appeal to some kind of finality: to power.

Most people immediately link power to its ultimate form: force. But the manifestations of physical power such as guns, war, violence, are used less often than covert forms of power, such as influence, control, direction. As Schermerhorn's comment suggests, since power is inherently scarce, it would appear that as one group obtains power, another loses it; one dominates and another is dominated.

Power within community is such a complex topic that it has dominated community literature in recent years. Community may be an equalizing association, in that all members belong. This is the root of the concept of 'citizen'. Yet, within most communities, both modern and traditional, some appear to belong more than others. In the case of voluntary membership, it may be that some wish to participate more and to give more emotionally and physically, receiving, in turn, more influence or authority. On the other hand, there are some communities in which some receive more than they give on the basis of elite status, strength, or skill that has no relationship to degrees of belonging.

Debates over the power of the group to curtail the rights of the individual and the power of one community over others, or between communities and other social collectivities, are abundant. This last concern is characteristic of the present era. Nisbet argues that community is a conservative concept: the powers of larger wholes – nations, states, or giant organizations – may be offset by the development of subunits such as communities. When churches or local governments or universities demand power prerogatives (e.g. tax exemptions), they do so in the name of the authority that the collective exercises over members. Nisbet's argument is that community, which is denounced as a radical threat to the *status quo*, is a tool of political conservatism.[17]

The range of authority or power in which community operates has been divided by Schneider into three categories: (1) the private as expressed in the family, (2) the cosmopolitan, as expressed by the state, and (3) the communal or public area.[18]

These views have been expressed in the classical sociological tradition by Emile Durkheim as follows:

> The Provincial spirit has disappeared never to return; the patriotism of the Parish has become an archaism that cannot be restored at will . . . Our activity is extended beyond those groups which are too narrow for it, and, moreover, a good deal of what happens there leaves us indifferent. There is thus produced a spontaneous weakening of the old social structure. Now, it is impossible for this organization to disappear without something replacing it . . . A nation can be maintained only if, between the State and the individual, there is intercalated a whole series of secondary groups

> near enough to the individuals to attract them strongly in their sphere of action and draft them, in this way, into the general torrent of social life.[19]

Community Power Structures

Political scientists tend to construct definitions of community more narrowly than sociologists, regarding it as that location legally defined in administrative units (e.g. the county, the state, the village). As the focus of political research moved away from the static and formal arrangements of structure to the dynamics of decision-making, it became clear that social factors were powerful indices of political behaviour. Knowing about voting, holding office, and passing laws did not guarantee that the operations of the political arena were understandable. As was clear in the study of politics in non-industrial societies where the various aspects of living are closely integrated, political processes are parts of wider cultural processes.

The recent literature on community power, however, is illuminating because it attempts to isolate communities (albeit legally determined units) and to relate structure, conflict, and power in these contexts. An example of how all three operate in a given situation might make this clearer. Although Hughes's study of a town in French Canada is not new, it brings the political and social elements of community dynamics together sharply.

French Canada in Transition: A Case Study

> For minority feeling is not so much a matter of number as of a felt disadvantage in some hierarchy, accompanied by the sense that strangers and strange institutions are wresting from one's people mastery over their own fates.
>
> *E. C. Hughes*[20]

Cantonville, a town in Quebec, Canada, has been described by Hughes as a frontier in which the French rural population meets with an industrialized town dominated by English industrial leaders. Rural communities, part of the tradition of French Canadians, are characterized by two potent institutions: the family and the parish. These two institutions are integrated 'with the larger society through colleges, hospitals, monasteries, convents, and seminaries'. The cultural orientation of both institutions and people was towards a rural past, for the provincial French Canadian had deep ties to the soil. Yet, he found himself in the town and an industrialized world controlled by the English 'outsiders'. The result was that the values and ideals he had adopted, and those expressed by the French Canadian spiritual and intellectual leaders have no connection with ordinary economic features in the life of the average Cantonville citizen. Hughes describes the plight of the French Canadian thus:

> Those who have been accustomed to state their values for them and those who guard their sacred symbols and sentiments have little authority over the bread and butter activities of the urban French Canadians. The kinds of knowledge and the personal qualities stressed by the intellectual leaders of French Canada do not coincide with those of the economic system in which most urban French Canadians have to work.[21]

Within the town of Cantonville, all political offices are controlled by French Canadians. All service industries, professional positions, service and local retail businesses are dominated by French Canadians. Almost all the social organizations (except the golf club, Chamber of Commerce, and Protestant religious groups) are completely maintained by the 90 per cent of the population that speaks French. Why then is it possible for an English minority to become so influential or to hold so much power?

The answer lies in the process of industrialization as it came to Cantonville. The French Canadian citizens of Quebec, like citizens of all colonial nations, found themselves living in the midst of an industrial revolution sponsored by outsiders. The outsiders, in this case the English, initiated and developed industries, using capital from sources outside the community, and operating under directions from headquarters that are also located 'outside'. Those English who migrate into Cantonville come to build, control, and maintain the industrial complex. However, the industries were staffed in all lower positions by French Canadians who had migrated from the farm into the town. Once in the town, the French Canadians become dependent for jobs upon industries managed by the English. Hughes explains the relationship in these words:

> The English population comes to perform specialized functions. It is, in short, a sort of new and specialized organ grafted into the local society.[22]

He argues that the function of the English in Quebec has been 'to create new points of activity to which the French Canadian population has rallied'.

The picture of Cantonville that emerges is of a French Canadian population held together by common religious and cultural ties but earning a living in industrial settings that are controlled by outsiders. Hughes sums the situation up in this way: 'The local and visible authority may be French Canadian, but the absent higher authority is English.'[23]

The English managerial elite justify their presence as industrial superiors by their conviction that the French Canadians have neither the expertise nor the interest to develop industrial operations. They argue that the close family ties among French Canadians would interfere with efficient operations in the plant and that it is essential to maintain English management to safeguard the capital investment, coordinate plant operations in Cantonville with the rest of the country, and ensure that modern managerial ideas are adopted. Although Hughes admits that the church-dominated educational system of the French Canadians is not well suited to produce industrial leaders and is, in fact, anti-industrial in outlook, he argues that there is probably sufficient talent among the Cantonville local population to assume high managerial positions if these opportunities were extended. However, it is unlikely that the English industrial leaders would relinquish their positions without a political struggle.

Hughes carefully detailed the many ways in which the two populations had contacts and differed – in recreational arrangements, educational institutions, and ceremonial life. The English did not participate in those parts of town life which provided the dominant concerns of the French Canadians: they have no leadership roles in the parish, never spoke out on political matters. As a result the English settlement 'lacks real liveliness and solidarity', and the French Canadian community was unable to play any part in the important spheres of industrial activity.

Cantonville is an example of the ways in which the essential political factors – structure, conflict, and power – interact. There was a viable social structure developed to sustain the French Canadian community. This maintained internal cohesion through the institutions of church and family, and gave direction to the lives of the rural-based population. But the community was unable to find the means of controlling the development of industrialization in the town, and was therefore powerless against the English managerial élite who directed the economic centres. Unlike the American or British experience, the people of Cantonville had not developed newer structures from which they could challenge industrial leadership, such as trade unions, trade associations, 'and other forms of interest groups which engage in conflict, bargaining and lobbying to maintain and improve the place of various estates in the economic and political world'.[24] Nor were the economic needs of the ordinary citizens recognized in the French Canadian educational system, or indeed, the entire cultural complex. French Canadian leaders were out of touch with the dilemmas that town living imposed upon Cantonville residents.

Thus in Cantonville one can see a French Canadian community challenged by industrial forces controlled by an élite not part of the community. The English settlement within the town provided a weak social union, creating only ineffectual social arrangements, since members were excluded from wider Cantonville concerns. Cantonville, the place, then, had two distinct social collectivities – the French Canadian and the English. Until those kinds of social structures developed which could deal with the problem of conflict between the two groups, it is unlikely that any kind of overall community would grow.

Hughes explains that Cantonville is typical of many communities faced with pressures that cannot be contained geographically and remain unaffected by any locally based authority. He notes:

> It has been a doctrine of our time that the earth's surface should be divisible into clearly bounded territories, each occupied by a racially and culturally homogeneous people who can celebrate their past, their present and their hopes in common ceremony and who can act together to administer their domestic affairs and to defend themselves from outside dangers. Few countries conform, in all particulars to this ideal.[25]

When members of communities find that they no longer control their destiny but are overwhelmed by forces more powerful than they are as individuals or as collectives – such as national or international industrialization, technological changes, mobility of peoples, ideas and institutions – they face a crisis of belief. One solution is to withdraw from the traditional community and join other, modified, social forms, or in the words of this discussion, build a new form of community. Another alternative is to find the political means of achieving power over outside pressures and restoring the authority that once belonged to the community. This alternative is the basis of many revolutionary confrontations, particularly in societies trying to modernize. The demand for power – *now* – from many different kinds of political group reflects the frustrations of helplessness. If the discontent and misery of the frustrated many is channelled into building political structures that can control and direct conflict, and give citizens a voice in the important realities of everyday life, it is possible that viable political communities will develop. If this does not happen, violence, revolution, and destruction may be the only means whereby such power can be obtained.

7 Community and commitment

Is it family writ large?

> For the young are, by their very nature, uncommitted. They constitute the only group who can perpetually renew its lack of commitment as its older members are siphoned off into the ranks of the committed.
>
> *P. Slater*[1]

The relationship between community and family is often misleading. Some view the community as an extension of the family, or an enlarged kinship unit. Traditionally, leaders of organizations dependent upon ideological support from participants (e.g. churches and schools) have found the family analogy useful. There is an emotional tone of warmth and security in the family image that is transferred to the wider association. It seems to be almost a 'natural' extension of loyalty to move from family to community; in some instances, it is a 'hierarchy' of identifications.

It is not coincidental that the family and the traditional community flourished in the same soil for so long. Both were held in fixed geographical and social space; both shared a loyalty to common values and standards of behaviour that fostered a homogeneous perspective. In return for group assistance to the family in the form of physical protection (laws and armies), group labour at harvest-time, assistance in floods and in other disasters, or even ritual condolences in grief, the community received back *from* the family loyalty. The family nourished the child's public development, teaching the young to accept those responsibilities imperative for communal functioning.

In spite of dramatic social changes in most societies, the family is still the important agent in determining patterns of commitment. The ways in which families shape personal values and guide development ultimately influence the ways in which the person creates a private view of the wider social world. But it is also true that other socializing agencies (e.g. school, peer groups) challenge familial monopoly, particularly as the structure of the traditional family is itself challenged.

VARIETIES OF FAMILY INFLUENCE

The nuclear family (that is, a unit composed of parents and unmarried offspring without other kin) in most fully industrialized societies has become the focus of many ambiguous relationships, confused expectations and uncertainties. One of the clearest indications of this confusion may be seen in terminological problems. For example, what do we call mother-in-law? Is she a relative (Mother? Grandmother?), or a friend (Jane?), or simply a third party (Mrs. Jones), or do we simply not call her anything.[2] More important, does the term 'family' apply only to the union of male and female and their offspring or can we apply it to two members of the same sex who adopt children, or groups of adults and children united by multiple marriages?[3] Just as it can be argued that the basis of community is gradually becoming a voluntary act of commitment and the selection among alternatives, belonging to a family may become a similar choice. And even as we ponder the name of the game and debate the rules, the game itself is being transformed before us. Control over reproduction is rapidly moving to events outside the family unit: to laboratories (e.g. test-tube babies); to political bodies (e.g. legislation to control overpopulation); and to economic conditions (e.g. the increase in women working, the availability of contraceptives).

Although it is obvious that the nuclear family is less independent as regards the socialization of its children, it is not clear how this directly affects the building of commitment mechanisms. The critical issue has been that of privatism. Critics of this type of family view it as a unit of consumption, as a tool of female exploitation, and as a fundamentally antisocial feature of capitalistic life because it defines values and goods in terms of the unit itself. Children are encouraged to seek individual rewards, private goals, and personal achievements. But the factors that lead to privatism are also those which lead to a permissiveness in child-care that reflects the tension between control and freedom found in child-rearing. Permissiveness, when it is not used as an epithet in the attack against 'lack of discipline', implies a recognition that the child has some freedom to act; it recognizes that there are elements of will and choice in development.[4] This does not mean that the child has a great range of alternatives: his dependency and lack of power restrict his options, as do the subtle forms of social control involving a manipulation of parent–child love and psychologically damaging kinds of behaviour so that 'each new recruit to the human race' will behave in 'substantially the same way as those who have already got here'.[5] But it does implant the notion that choices can be made, even if one argues that: (a) the choices are fraudulent and real alternatives do not exist, or (b) the immaturity of the child precludes an ability to choose wisely.

Contrasted to the recognition that a child may, in certain instances, give or withdraw his participation or agreement in certain matters, is the belief that child-rearing must be totally prescribed and regulated. Ever since Plato's republican idyll presented a plan by which children were cared for in community institutions rather than private families, reformers have been fascinated by the potentialities of child-care in new and more revolutionary forms. Most of the programmes have not lasted long or have been meagrely researched; few have been successful when the other dominant social forms have been well entrenched in a given society. Consequently the kibbutz was greeted eagerly by many social scientists as an exciting laboratory in which to investigate this philosophy.[6]

Within the kibbutz, children are reared together from birth by professional childminders. Parents may see their children daily for a few hours, but they are not encouraged to separate the child from his peer community. The children eat, sleep, study, and play in their own living-quarters, and the parents remain in distinct units.

Most observers have noted the strength of the kibbutz in the fair treatment given to the children. They develop fewer feelings of jealousy and anger towards others, are healthy, well-educated, law-abiding, and devoted to the service of Israel. But Bruno Bettleheim has pointed out that the strength of group life has also diminished originality and autonomy, the necessary ingredients in creativity.[7] The kibbutz, in many ways, is a microcosm of the deep tensions between individual and group which are manifest in a community. In order to give most completely of oneself, one must surrender that which is most precious:

individuality. But if one gives all one's individuality, one is no longer as rich and valuable as the participant who has retained something of himself. If the end requires a group dependent upon strong individual units, the group is weakened by an excess of individuality and by its opposite oversocialization.

SIGNIFICANCE OF FAMILY VARIATIONS

Much of the social energies of the individual during his lifetime are devoted to maintaining the tension between himself and the community. The kibbutz child, unlike the child in the nuclear family, is less aware of the tension because he has been trained to put communal factors above his private concerns. The important aspects of child-training are questions of priority. The kibbutz child is guided to make a total commitment to the community, whereas the other arrangement leads to only a partial commitment. In the nuclear family, there is a constant adjustment between person and collective, creating a tension that has been the source of much creative energy. It has also been the basis of persecution for minorities and dissenters. At its best, it has stimulated thoughtful, willing commitment to collectivities, given because the person finds more satisfaction within community than outside. At its worst, it fosters the excesses of repression.

During the past few years there has been a widespread revival of the ancient idea of commune families. These are deliberate attempts to modify the isolation of the nuclear family and to encourage more diffuse commitment in terms of human relationships. In some cases, the child has many parents and the degree of involvement with social worlds outside the commune is minimal; but in others, the commune represents a variation of family life in which participants continue to operate outside the group. The varieties in number, style, permanence, and goals among communes is impressive, but the popularity and potency of the movements attest to the concern with providing alternatives to family life as it is now constituted.[8]

Research in child-rearing practices among different social classes has also suggested ways in which varieties of training influence later commitment. For example, lower-class families may have the effect of stimulating peer-group communities more quickly than do middle-class pressures upon the child to achieve individually. Personality factors are also important: some individuals are more 'open' to others and enjoy social situations; some families are more open to contact with non-family persons. There are important cultural differences that influence family habits. In some societies the dominant ideology requires that the family 'looks to its own', and 'minds its own business', whereas in others families are encouraged to lean towards public groupings. Finally, there are different familial forms and social arrangements that influence the child's understanding of community demands.[9]

Another important element in determining the family's role in the early stages of community development is the role of the government. Wherever the family has been a powerful centre of human activities, governments, particularly those expanding their political control, have attempted to break its authority. The fundamental ideological conflict between the Chinese family and the Communist regime, for example, has demonstrated this vividly.[10]

What is interesting at this stage of history is the approach to community from the opposite ends of the ideological spectrum. In the West, men are seeking communities to counteract loneliness, lack of power, and the emotional difficulties of personal problems: they move from the personal to the collective. Within China and other socialist states, the purges, the trials of intellectuals, and the military pressures on satellite countries reflect the need of individuals to withdraw from total commitment to preserve some individuality from the whole. These sweeping trends, however, do not preclude the social fact that many ordinary persons in both kinds of society seek means to harmonize their conflicts. It is quite likely that just as I, a Western sociologist, seek evidence of existing community in many different kinds of social forms, Communist writers are documenting the many ways in which individuals are preserving their privacy in the midst of group demands.

COMMITMENT AND COMMUNITY

Since modern communities are based increasingly upon selection by membership, the means by which the individual commits himself to the collective is important. Etzioni reminds us that commitment is a positive involvement, the opposite of alienation. It is the active ingredient in any community, requiring the individual to invest both emotional and physical energy in social structures outside his immediate personal milieu.[11]

Like many important words, it is difficult to define commitment. Some members accept all communal norms and participate fully in community processes, whereas others are peripherally concerned, ranging in Toch's words from 'faith to fanaticism'.[12] A religious order requires a member to renounce other ties, break radically with his past, and belong exclusively to the order. A university demands a strong commitment from students for a selected period of time, but cannot demand the exclusive preoccupation that is found in the religious order. In many kinds of modern communities, it is likely that members are committed for only a limited period of time, belonging to different kinds of communities at different stages in life.

Because commitment to a modern community is seldom total, many claim that it is of little consequence. However, community by its very nature demands a substantial emotional and physical investment and represents a significant expenditure of human resources. As a social form, community membership encompasses many demands upon the members' social capital, even if it is likely that there is 'some money in the bank' remaining. As a matter of fact, the monetary analogy is quite useful. The individual who scatters his social resources too widely will not receive sufficient return from his investments to receive satisfactory communal returns, such as 'belonging', 'recognition', or 'acceptance'. It seems logical to assume that most social actors soon learn how to manage their social investments so as to receive some returns. Unfortunately, this has been a very neglected area of social research and social scientists have not been particularly interested in commitment mechanisms. Our fascination with the social problems of the system – disease and pathology – has kept us from examining those devices which men have found useful in developing loyalty to wider associations. The role of the family in influencing children's attitudes in this area has never been systematically investigated.

Kanter has suggested that the foundations of commitment are threefold.[13] The first is long-sustained, continuous commitment that is based upon cognitive orientations: the person sees the advantages of belonging. Another kind is identified by cohesion: commitment is based upon the formation of positive emotional ties and one can sense some satisfaction from belonging: it is fun to belong. A third type is based upon obedience and the decision by the member that community demands are legitimate and authorized: he 'should belong'.

In describing the process of commitment in Pentecostal and Black Power Movements, Gerlach and Hine view it as a psycho-social state that results from an identity-altering experience.[14] It would seem that in many cases, commitment to a community is based upon a need for maintenance of identity. This also raises important questions about the ways in which commitment is sustained: the rewards, so to speak, of communities. For example, Reiss calls attention to the status-conferring properties of community,[15] an important factor in developing sustained commitment.

FAMILY, COMMUNITY, AND COMMITMENT

The community shares with the family certain affective characteristics; the family is important in developing both the conscious and the will to belong to a community. Like community, the family has been attacked on the basis of many superficial criticisms. Some research suggests that the isolation of the nuclear family is not as total as many believe, contact with kin, perhaps different in form, is still a significant feature of family life. Grandmother may not live with the family, but she comes for visits, telephones, writes, sends assistance in the form of money and in other ways. Geographical proximity is not a requirement for many kinds of interaction.[16] Likewise, many elderly people find satisfaction and pleasure from independence that cannot be obtained within the kinship unit. In other words, before we despair of family arrangements completely, we must not accept a totally bleak accounting of developments.

Technology has given the young a status that is unique. Slater compares it to the advantages of the American youth in a frontier society and in immigrant movements, both of which favoured those who were physically stronger, more adaptable, and less conditioned to the past.[17] Mead goes further when she writes:

> Today, nowhere in the world are there elders who know what the children know, no matter how remote and simple the societies are in which the children live. In the past there were always some elders who knew more than any children in terms of their experience of having grown up with a cultural system. Today it is not

> only that the parents are no longer guides but that there are no guides, whether one seeks them in one's own country or abroad. There are no elders who know what those who have been reared within the last twenty years know about the world into which they were born.[18]

Under such conditions it would be difficult to teach the child commitment to a fixed community: he will find his loyalties via many routes. It is unlikely that he will become totally committed to any community, except for brief periods of time. His will be a partial and limited commitment, withdrawn or given on many different grounds. Such developments may appear disturbing – and to those who seek the kind of emotional stability and permanence in community they want to find in the family, they will be frightening. But we must remind ourselves that the challenge of reality is in the attempt, the venture – and the hope.

8 Organizations and social bonds

Is community a stage?

> Just as modern chemistry concerns itself with what it calls the chemical bond, seeking the forces that make atoms stick together as molecules, so does sociology investigate the forces that enable biologically derived human beings to stick together from the moment, quite literally, of their conception.
>
> *Robert Nisbet*[1]

Our understanding of social bonding is less than that of the chemist's knowledge of chemical bonding, yet it is urgent that we attempt to study what forces bring men to each other and into wider social systems. Nisbet's terminology may be current but the relationships to which he refers are the familiar Durkheimian issues of social order and the ancient Aristotelian questions regarding man's nature.[2]

It is evident that bonds between persons are multiple – some are based upon biological factors, such as sex, stage of life, or age; some are historically and culturally determined. We know very little about the components of social bonds and how they differ in various social structures. Tiger talks of bonding as a biological process, 'the outcome of which involves specific individuals recognizing other individuals as directly and distinctly relevant to themselves'.[3] But, most relevant to our discussion of community, we have not been able to determine the qualitative importance and variations between different social linkages.

Because modern man can voluntarily select his communities to a degree not possible in the past, his choices must rest upon some evaluative foundations. In the absence of many empirical studies, it seems reasonable to suggest that one criterion would be pleasure or satisfaction derived from participating in social relationships. Since community, wherever found, represents men interacting together on many levels – physical, emotional, instrumental, expressive – communal membership must be satisfying on many levels of experience and must involve emotional and physical investments and returns.

To say that the communal bond is both emotional and instrumental may be another way of saying that it reflects elements of 'positive concern'. This has been defined by sociologist Bert Adams as including: obligation and need, long-term involvement, continuing interest, and a positive affectional factor.[4] When positive concern grows less, ties weaken. Or stated another way, the social bond found in community is inherently personal; commitment may have many roots but one of these includes an identification with other human beings.

Social bonds are found in every collectivity and often it is impossible to disentangle different kinds of bonds. In an effort to understand the strength and significance of communal bonds, it might be valuable to examine bonding in another context, for often in the process of determining what is not related, we begin to understand what is related. The choice of bonding in organizations is based upon several factors: organizations are one of the most pervasive and powerful social forms to be found in technologically advanced societies. Frequently, organizational bonds are so embracing that they appear to be replacing communal bonds, and it is clear that the two kinds of social form come close together at times. However, because of a fundamental difference in the basis of the bond, the two are not interchangeable and efforts to replace communal bonds with organizational ties lead to serious consequences in terms of social satisfaction.

MODERN ORGANIZATIONS

> The journey to work is the great architect of urban structure; and now (for almost everyone) means 'work' in an organization.
>
> *W. J. Mackenzie*[5]

Organizations are brought into existence because they can achieve specific goals, but the number and variety of organizations are so great that it is difficult to determine which goals are receiving priority, which are in competition with each other; if new goals are added and others changed; and whether the stated goals are, in fact, being accomplished. One problem with studying organizations in this way is that it directs attention towards the formal arrangements of structure and does not deal with the dynamics of individuals working together.[6] The popularity of the goals approach, or systems analysis, is that it relates organizations to other parts of society and enables one to see the ways in which different parts of society affect one another, raising issues of priority, effectiveness, and personal participation. The problem of accountability, particularly in regard to non-economic factors in organizational development, leads to important political and social questions which are beyond the scope of this discussion. But the understanding of the functional nature of organizations is pertinent to an understanding of the instrumental ties which characterizes membership, as opposed to the more inclusive bonds of a community.

This is not to argue that communal bonds are not also instrumental. In the past, particularly in the geographical community of place, these bonds were so obvious that the threat of banishment – the most severe form of punishment and an extreme sanction – was poised as the ultimate threat to the member. From the opposite perspective, however, well-established communities generally create elaborate rituals to stress that belonging is a result of 'being' and not necessarily the consequence of 'doing', although the two are closely related. For example, anthropologist Victor Turner suggests that *rites de passage* present us with a 'moment in and out of time' and:

> . . . in and out of secular social structure, which reveals, however fleetingly, some recognition (in symbol if not always in language) of a generalized social bond that has ceased to be and has simultaneously yet to be fragmented into a multiplicity of structural ties.[7]

Although the social ties within an organization are predominantly instrumental, they are not as direct and clear as logic would dictate. Many organizations, for a variety of reasons, have adopted some communal characteristics. Elaborate insurance plans, health centres, canteen facilities, sports grounds, and real-estate ventures have emerged as areas of occupational interest. Some firms adopt the theme that 'this is a good place to work' by stressing the positive aspects of the enterprise. 'Good management techniques', incentives for developing a 'team' approach, and even the official recognition of unions as the institutionalized acknowledgment that conflict is inherent in long-sustained social relationships, stimulate a community-like atmosphere.

Many organizations attempt to create the appearance of community by symbolic manipulation. For example, among white-collar employees, the organization presents a message of 'concern'. Personnel advertisements invite applicants to 'join' an organization that 'cares'. These appeals have relevance to many in modern society who define themselves through work, and job satisfaction includes a wide range of factors besides the specific task. As Whyte suggests, the so-called 'organization man' doesn't just work for an organization, but belongs to it and subscribes to a social ethic that justifies his place in the organization and its dominance over other life activities.[8] Classical Marxian theory is most relevant to this area of instrumental bonding and one way in which it can be demonstrated is in the severance of instrumental ties during periods of lay-off.

THE END OF THE COMMUNAL MYTH

A reduction in personnel – the lay-off – has both personal and social consequences. Those members of an organization who view it in normative terms, and are rewarded in terms of prestige and status, are more likely to be persuaded that the organization has communal characteristics, and are, therefore, likely to be more affected psychologically by a lay-off than those who have not held such illusions. Psychological rejection may be less severe when an entire plant or industry, such as mining, is run down, because these cases can be interpreted more directly as a result of impersonal forces. But even here the individual in his private life suffers despair and loss of status. It matters little that the redundancy was not caused by personal failings if the effect is to disturb the individual's self-esteem, and even impersonal criteria for selecting men (seniority and plant task) may be bitterly resented by the very people the procedure was designed to protect.

When the lay-off is imminent, power relationships within the organization become discernible and employees recognize that they have little ability to change decisions. Those with the highest expectations suffer the most disillusionment as the communal image is rudely shattered.

An interesting documentation of the physical deterioration which accompanies this psychological process is found in Alfred Slote's detailed study of a paint plant which closed in Detroit, Michigan. During the two years that elapsed between the announcement that the plant would close and the actual event, all personnel involved showed measurable physical and mental strain in the form of illness.[9]

The organizational bond remains an instrumental bond, in spite of being tempered by unions, law, and society in general. The communal bond, on the other hand, must be more than a functional tie because it involves concerns with the affective aspects of the individual's life: his identity, his commitment to the collective, and his emotional well-being. As Arensberg and Kimball argue, what distinguishes communities from other associations is 'their wholeness and inclusiveness'.[10]

MULTIPLE BONDING

Although redundancy reveals how fragile are organizational ties of positive concern, there are several conditions of contemporary society that suggest that the bonds of community and organization will become more entwined. As complexity increases, multiple bonding is likely to become part of the organizational scene, not only from the perspective of the organization, but also from that of the employee. This is based upon the assumption that bureaucratic arrangements are no longer satisfactory in post-industrial society. Under conditions of instability, the major condition of organizational survival is rapid adaptation to change, and, for this, the ponderous bureaucratic machinery serves only as a stumbling-block. Participants have a vested interest in maintaining a private niche in the organization, and even if adherence to strict procedures ('following the book') causes delay and inefficiency, the desire to protect individual territories is more pressing.

The growing recognition that the human factor in organization is critical, not because of employee welfare (although from some perspectives, this is paramount), but because the organizational process is dependent upon human resources, has been summarized by Katz and Kahn:

> The formal hierarchical organization is an instrument of great effectiveness: it offers great economies over unorganized effort: it

> achieves great utility and compliance. But its deficiencies include great waste of human potential for innovation and creativity and great psychological cost to members, many of whom spend their lives in organizations without caring much either for the system (except its intrinsic rewards and accidental impersonal relationships) or the goal toward which the system is redirected. The modification of hierarchical organization to meet these criticisms is one of the great needs of human life.[11]

One of the difficulties of understanding organizational dynamics is to be found in the analysis of the organization from the perspective of goals or external criteria, and to understand what participants in the organization actually adopt as objectives. According to Burns and Stalker:

> . . . men and women do not ordinarily yield themselves wholly to use as resources by others; indeed, to do so infringes the human purpose of controlling the situation confronting the individual. In every organized working community, therefore (except those for which religious zeal, political enthusiasm, or some other dedication of the self identifies the personal ends of its members with those they believe to be pursued by the others or by their leader), individuals seek to realize other purposes than those they recognize as the organization's.[12]

There is also a psychological change that is having a strong impact upon organizational development. How deep and strong the revolt is against technology in all its forms, particularly among the young, may be debated; but the widespread distaste and vocal disatisfaction expressed by many with distinct organizational patterns can no longer be ignored in terms of recruitment, personnel development, and long-range commitment to organizational objectives.[13]

THE DANGERS OF CONFUSING DIFFERENT TYPES OF BOND

There is a danger of confusing social bonds based upon functional requirements with those based upon expressive ties, particularly when the vocabulary of positive concern is co-opted by many. The social consequences of continual deception are the loss of trust and the reluctance to commit oneself to wider public collectives. For this reason, Lionel Trilling argues that: 'One of the most salient characteristics of the culture of our time is the intense, we might say obsessive, concern with authenticity as a quality of personal life and as a criterion of art.'[14] One of the ways in which members of a community avoid this play upon authenticity is the recognition (sometimes without conscious awareness) that they have a common destiny. Since their ties are grounded upon positive personal concerns, there is a social responsibility in a community which cannot be overlooked. As noted earlier in the discussion, unlike a group, community demands an ethic of concern; a structured commonality which encourages a social conscience towards others. This is why Delespesse defines community as:

> . . . an organic and stable fraternal association of persons accepting the responsibility for one another, through sharing both what they are and what they have, in order to bring about the union of mankind.[15]

The requirements for expressive ties within a communal context makes such a definition more than idealism or hope.

THE LIMITS OF BONDING: RETICULATION

The concept of social bonding can be carried too far. Some would consider our ties to collectives to be more like fine threads that criss-cross and break easily. For example, Gerlach and Hine have adopted the term 'reticulation' to describe the kinds of bonds that are developed within the Pentecostal and Black Power movements. Pointing out that reticulate refers to something that is weblike, resembling a network with crossing and intercrossing lines, they use the term:

> . . . to describe an organization in which the cells, or nodes are tied together, not through any central point, but rather through intersecting sets of personal relationships and other group linkages.[16]

They found that social ties were based upon personal relationships between members, by the activities of travelling evangelists or spokesmen, and by certain basic ideological themes. In this instance, reticulation enabled the association to be adaptive and permitted the maximum penetration of people and ideas. In most modern communities, reticulation provides a more accurate description of social ties than does bonding.

Another significant limitation on bonding is the requirement for recognition of the bonds rather than the strength of these. Nisbet points out that it is neither numbers nor commonness, but the conscious recognition of sharing, that is critical.

> Tribe, clan, nation, business enterprise, church, family, mutual aid association, criminal conspiracy, town, social class, play group, gang, neighbourhood – each of these is a social aggregate for the reason just given – each is composed of members – however far flung in area they may be – who either directly or indirectly through common symbols, are aware of each other and are influenced by each other.[17]

A third criticism of bonding is that the use of concepts such as positive concern and emotional satisfaction evoke sentimental, rather than realistic, images of human association. But as Greeley has pointed out, this may not be so, and can, in fact, lead to the Hobbesian question: what makes society possible? He suggests that: 'The laws, the conventions, the mores that hold us together in the human community are nothing more than a thin red line we use to hold terror at bay.'[18] Greeley proposes friendship as one attempt to 'transcend the boundaries of terror'. The social bonding found in community may simply be an organized effort to find social supports to avoid the abyss of being human. But whatever the cause, the communal bond – or the 'ties' – are personal, inclusive, and emotionally tinged.

A SOCIOLOGICAL NOTE

In an age of slogans, terms like 'the quality of life' can become meaningless. To determine empirical referents for such words is difficult, but important. We know that some types of social bond are more satisfying and are valued more highly than others; some last longer and are expressed more directly, individually, and completely than others. If there is any value in the study of community, it is with these 'intangible' aspects of interaction. Terms like commitment, dedication, authenticity, and positive concern can be slippery to work with in specific research situations. But it is a respectable and necessary sociological task to relate personal goals to reality; stated beliefs to practice: ordinary social understandings to social structures. Unfortunately, measuring has often become an exercise in unmasking or in irony. The 'games people play' are fascinating, and well worth sociological study, but we deceive ourselves if we do not recognize that we all play games of some sort. The reasons why we play – to survive, to enjoy, to win – are also the proper concerns of sociology, In a pluralistic environment, one in which voluntary membership increasingly makes individual choice possible, problems of measurement, identification, and interpretation of values are difficult. But to remain aloof from such problems is to deny the most important aspects of human existence.[19]

Because community deals with values, it has remained a central sociological problem throughout history, and will remain important. Saying this does not mean that we cannot examine all human associations critically, empirically, and scientifically. Nor is this a conservative and static view of social behaviours because it expresses an interest in social structures.[20] Studying community is based upon the view that sociology must be concerned with the total human experience and the organization of such experience in all social forms.

To be interested in others, to be concerned, are more than moral attributes; they are the essence of life, psychologically and sociologically. Without these, nothing remains. As expressed by Weston LaBarre:

> Basic problems in our day are less objective-scientific than subjective-moral ones. In the scientific method we already have an effective way of solving problems, of understanding and making things. Politico-economic and social ills derive from moral failures in the using and sharing of things. Indeed, murderously competing dogmas of how to do this actually constitute the most real danger to mankind, in a new round of religious wars, the politico-economic ones of our day. In science we are willing to make experiments to uncover facts: in morals we are not.[21]

9 Social roles and institutions

Is community love?

At a meeting of the faculty of a certain large university, a proposal for a new administrative policy was being discussed. The debate was long and intense before a final vote of adoption was taken. As the professors filed out of the room an instructor continued the discussion with one of the older deans.

'Well' observed the latter official, 'it may be a little hard on some people; but I feel sure that, in the long run, the new plan will be for the best interests of the institution.'

'Do you mean that it will be good for the students?' inquired the younger man.

'No', the dean replied, 'I mean it will be for the good of the whole institution.'

'Oh, you mean that it will benefit the faculty as well as the students?'

'No', said the dean, a little annoyed. 'I don't mean that; I mean it will be a good thing for the institution itself.'

'Perhaps you mean the trustees then – or the Chancellor?'

'No, I mean the institution, the *institution*! Young man, don't you know what an institution is?'

Floyd Allport[1]

Mackenzie has called institutions 'social facts which change relatively slowly'.[2] By this he means that institutions are made up of all the people, behaviours, and ways by which any given society arranges the fundamental concerns of life: economics, education, religion, etc. Persons play parts in the institution: they 'perform' roles, the role being the sum total of expectations and behaviours.

Institutional analysis is particularly concerned with understanding the ways in which social roles develop, change, and operate. Every major institution depends upon the smooth functioning of persons in their role capacities to behave along patterned and prescribed lines. Thus, in Floyd Allport's story, the young man was astutely correct in trying to define the effects of the decision upon specific role-players, i.e. students, faculty, or trustees. The dean, on the other hand, had adopted a commonly held assumption that the institution represents more than the sum of the individual parts, and is a form of social reality in itself.

INSTITUTION OR COMMUNITY

A basic difference between an institution and a community centres upon the concept of roles. In a community the member is not viewed as a specialist or as a performer who assumes certain tasks. Rather, the community is the context in which the person *may* be seen as a complete unity. For example, a teacher plays a particular role in the educational institution. He is expected to act in a predictable manner deemed suitable for teachers. Within a given society, a teacher may be recognized by what he does and how he acts in the educational system. The teacher who belongs to a community, however, seeks in this context the opportunity to view himself not only as a teacher, but also as a husband, a father, a part-time artist, a middle-class wage-earner, an Englishman, an Anglican. He does not have to play a specific role in the community, but can just 'be'. Moreover, he is accepted in a community on the basis of 'being'.[3]

This oversimplification tends to make the distinctions between institutional and communal forms much sharper than they really are in every-day life. One reason for the blurring of forms is that man's freedom to select among many alternatives usually leads to questions of *priorities*. As emphasized earlier, we seldom find a member totally committed to his community, any more than we find people completely identified with their role in an institution. Rather, modern man gives more or less priority to one social form in his life at any given time, and generally is a member of many organizations, institutions, and a community simultaneously.[4]

For example, the teacher is part of an educational institution. It is possible, although unlikely, that the school may also be a community, in which the teacher can be totally involved in all his roles. But, more typically, the teacher finds himself as an integer in an institutional setting and also as a member of another community. In a community the person is both an emotional and a physical being, so that the satisfaction of communal membership is found partly in this aspect of personal wholeness and unity, resulting from lack of specialization. Schneider expresses the distinction by arguing that the community member is always the amateur and never the professional in his communal context. He writes:

> The professional's supremacy is with his skill, the amateur's with his spirit, and community is preeminently the place for expressions of the human spirit.[5]

Schneider argues that the skills of professionals are for sale – but the amateur gives his in return for appreciation or honour – communal gifts; likewise, the amateur uses institutions to achieve personal ends whereas the professional adopts institutional goals as his own.

THE ATTACK AGAINST INSTITUTIONS

Particular roles are usually played in settings. Goffman calls these 'social establishments' and defines them as 'any place surrounded by fixed barriers to perception in which a particular kind of activity regularly takes place'.[6] According to Illich, performing roles in these specific settings leads to a kind of 'institutional wisdom' which actually perverts professions by packaging roles. Because we have established hospitals, for example, we have made it increasingly difficult to attend to the sick at home, and we have made the doctor dependent upon the facilities of the hospital to perform his role. We have made teachers dependent upon schools, lawyers upon courts, clergy upon churches. This leads, in Illich's view, 'inevitably to physical pollution, social polarization, and psychological impotence: three dimensions in a process of global degradation and modernized misery'.[7] He also develops an institutional spectrum ranging from those which are convivial (distinguished by spontaneous use) to those which are manipulative (require unwilling consumption). He explains:

> At both extremes of the spectrum we find service institutions, but on the right the service is imposed manipulation, and the client is made the victim of advertising, aggression, indoctrination, im-

> prisonment, or electroshock. On the left the service is amplified opportunity within formally defined limits, while the client remains a free agent.[8]

Most modern institutions tend to be right wing in the sense that they are complex, costly, and try to convince the consumer that he requires the help of the institution. Most left-wing institutions become, in terms of our discussion, more community-like. The community doctor, for example, may be contrasted with the surgeon on a scale of specificity within his profession.

Frankenberg,[9] in fact, has developed a continuum role of analysis using audience overlap as one of several indices of a rural–urban continuum, arguing that 'complexity' changes to 'complication' as technological division of labour increases.

THE DANGERS AND ATTRACTIONS OF ROLE SIMPLIFICATION

The difficulties created by role specialization have led many to adopt community as a form of 'back to nature' – the solution to complexity. It leads critics of institutions to Illich's position: namely, the abolition of institutions because they have become obstacles to the performance of the very tasks for which they were created. As Michael Shanks concluded in his contemplation of the decade of the sixties, 'resistance to change seems to have strengthened in our society'.[10] It has seemed almost impossible to make institutional reforms of sufficient magnitude to change values, so that debates over the 'quality of life' usually begin with efforts to bypass traditional institutional arrangements.

Nor is it puzzling why institutions remain fixed. By formalizing roles and standardizing procedures, they appear to remain stable. According to Schon, this helps us to reduce uncertainty and provides a strategy for dealing with change in other areas of life.[11] Just as we wish to anchor our identities within specific, definable communities, so we wish to regulate basic life activities by controlling institutional processes. Unfortunately, it cannot succeed because institutions must respond to change or they become both irrelevant and inefficient.

There is an urgent need for a new style in role performance: a style of simplicity and directness. In many ways this style is in conflict with the professionalism we have fostered in the past twenty years. The latter is based upon penetrating and skilful specialization, objective evaluation, and role-playing within institutional settings. The new style of simplicity is related to – but not inherently a part of – communal structures. It diminishes rather than enlarges role distance;[12] it is less bureaucratic, less impersonal, and more generalized.

Goode[13] suggests that the tension within role-playing may be the source of developing this new style. For example, as the individual reorders priorities and changes habits, bargains between various roles, and allocates his resources to performances differently, he in fact alters his entire life-style.

Community provides a stage in which the individual may seek personal integration, But, more important, it may be a way of organizing roles to encompass a wider perspective. For example, the movement to organize health services on the basis of local areas, rather than dividing medical care among several institutions, may do this. This is the idea behind 'community care' for the mentally ill, and the efforts to coordinate several different agencies working together. (In actual practice, however, community care has often become a synonym for doing nothing: e.g. for returning the problem of the mentally ill patient back to his family.)[14] Another example is found in the desire for 'community control of schools, and is advocated by many minority groups who are disatisfied with the present institutionalized arrangements. These movements can be interpreted as efforts to make institutions more 'community-like'.

SOCIETAL AND PERSONAL INTEGRATION

Because community deals with the person as a whole and can thereby provide a context for integration, it does not follow that communities can develop societal integration. In fact, as the number and variety of communities increase in modern life, it may appear that the larger human aggregates of state and nation will become less consistent, monolithic, and stable. The questions of levels of integration are profoundly significant political topics. If social man must develop communal structures to survive, and if we must also maintain superstructures to preserve order, arbitrating between competing social demands and organizing the allocation of resources in a complex technological environment, the development of multiple, intersecting, temporary, and non-permanent social structures – the kind of modern communities we have been seeking – is necessary.

In this sense, roles are not abolished, as many primitive communitarians would suggest, or fully integrated to eliminate specialization; but are modified, changed, and shifted in the light of new demands. One of the ironies of the renewed interest in community is that so deep are the fears of breakdown that any suspicion of difference is seen as a threat. In a discussion of 'paradise now' John Passmore writes:

> The young are rebelling, in part, against the atomistic tendencies of modern society. But they have reacted, in a manner only too typical of human beings, by reverting to the old perfectionalist – and in the end tyrannical – ideal of a total unity rather than the admittedly more complex ideal of a plurality of intersecting communities. It is very natural to argue thus: the experience of belonging to a community is essential to 'humanity', therefore, the best of all possible worlds would be a total community to which everyone would belong.[15]

A total community would be so devoid of personal expression and so rigid that it could not provide the context for either integration – both personal or group – or development. In short, it would cease to be a community, for it could no longer remain the stage on which man 'becomes'.

ROLE COMMUNITIES

Goode has suggested that professions themselves constitute a community in which members share an identity, agree upon role definitions, speak a common language, share common values, assume some permanent membership status, and understand the social boundaries within which they operate. By sharing a function and developing patterns by which members operate together, professions, in fact, constitute a new form of community.[16]

We frequently refer to institutions and community, e.g. school *and* community, clinic *and* community, church *and* community. But as we begin to transform institutions, we recognize how meaningless the 'and' is in any practical relationship. The President of an American college noted that there is not one community and the college, but many; and that these communities are part of the institution and vice versa.[17] If we apply Goffman's insight regarding total institutions – those which contain within themselves all the necessary ingredients for life activities (e.g. hospitals, prisons) – we see that total institutions are social hybrids, combining elements characteristic of organizations and communities of place.[18]

It is conceivable that in this evolution the cross-breeding between communal and institutional elements will add to the crisis affecting all social institutions – literally, their complete breakdown in the face of change and complexity. The alternative would be the development of sets of relationships that encompass a wider field of activity, based not upon the performance of roles within a setting, but upon the solution of tasks that are designated as communal problems. In the work of community development, the major aim is to 'influence linkages between arenas', or to relate various role-responsibilities towards specific issues and social change.[19] It is what Arensberg and Kimball refer to as the 'fit between attitude and behavior, a belief and a cultural pattern, an institutional norm and a custom or sanction'.[20] Cross-breeding of forms will make role-players less specialized because they will have a multiplicity of goals, a mixed audience of other professionals, political leaders, and general members, and, most important, a recognition that the institutional and communal stages are not categorically separate.

TERMINOLOGICAL CONFUSION

The discussion so far may suggest that there are precise differences between communities, institutions, groups, and organizations. In everyday life these distinctions are not sharp. Although these provide us with useful analytical tools, they distort investigation by making differences appear more clear-cut than they are. Individuals participate in all four forms, and it may be helpful to look briefly at these:

Social Form	*Characteristics*
Primary groups	small, face-to-face interaction: unspecialized. Example: family.
Organizations	large number of parts, official goals, formal structure, divided by specialities into parts. Example: General Motors.
Institutions	national in scope or coterminous with entire society; functions which may be subdivided into organizations and groups. Example: the economic system.

Communities	unspecialized; presonal; integrative context. Example: religious order.

An organization the size of General Motors, in some ways (e.g. Gross National Product, capital investment, and monthly payroll accounts) might be larger and more complex than the total economic system of some small nations.

The criterion of size cannot differentiate these. Role behaviour suggests a more effective approach because the concept of role leads one to a consideration of the role-player, thereby introducing the human component into the discussion. As I will suggest in the next chapter, it is this focus upon human beings which is critical in considering community.

10 Social networks and choice

Is community talk?

> To learn to be human is to develop through the give and take of communication an effective sense of being an individually distinctive member of a community; one who understands and appreciates its beliefs, desires and methods, and who contributes to a further conversion of organic powers into human resources and values.
>
> *John Dewey*[1]

John Dewey recognized that communication is at the heart of any community: we can only share in common what we can communicate with others. Communication – the process of receiving and sending messages – is, fact, the life-blood of all social structures. One political scientist, Karl Deutsch, suggests that it is the nervous system of the body politic, in line with the 'muscles and bones' metaphor used by social scientists.[2] Sociologically speaking, communication is the means by which the shared perspectives of the group, the agreed-upon understandings that permit existence, bind men to each other, reflect current social behaviour, and actually mould future actions.

All collectivities have some recognized channels of communication. But today we face new problems. The sheer quantity of information sent out by means of steadily improving technological instruments, and the increase in the number of channels from which men may select messages, is overwhelming. In the past, because they were isolated and self-sufficient social centres, communities provided effective screening devices to insulate members against conflicting and unrelated messages from outside. As these conditions have vanished, it has become impossible for communities to exclude other messages completely, although

I would like to suggest that modern forms of community still serve as clearing houses in which messages that are non-related or out of tune with the communal belief system are discarded. One method of sorting is by sending messages along private and personal channels that overlap at some points, which is basically the concept of social networks adopted in this discussion as a possible step in locating modern communities.

Sociologists have recognized the significance of communication channels in studying communities as an important means of discovering social structure. For example, when we began to understand who has access to various channels, we come close to the foundations of power relationships among members. Furthermore, differences in communication styles between members often illustrate patterns of subordination and dominance, and explain many subtleties of influence management. Educators, as noted before, are recognizing how pervasive speech codes are in the development of thought and the manipulation of ideas. The symbolic meanings of group understandings and values have provided researchers with insight into the dimensions of group experience that serve integrative social functions.

One important area of communications that has been of great importance in discussions of modern community is that of the mass media, for the development of mechanical instruments is uniquely a feature of modern societies, reflecting and influencing their changes in scale, complexity, and technological invention. There has been a long sustained controversy among contemporary observers concerning the link between the media and the creation of life-styles and social forms.

According to Aranguren, technology has already changed speech-styles, so that the language of older people is characterized by messages that can be seen 'coming a long way off, arrive in leisurely fashion, and have become redundant to a good listener before the message is finished'. He argues that the language of the young – or new language – is elliptic and allusive, transmitting messages that are condensed and full of unspoken implications, so that it 'is difficult for someone who does not belong to the same peer group to grasp it'. He adds:

> There are other cases when it is not so much the language that has aged as the linguistic code, the 'key' to the cipher: the old words have been divorced from their usual context and even their

accepted meaning, to be put into a completely new situation and given fresh significance.[3]

Because language is the foundation of culture, the use of speech codes can define effective communal boundaries, as historically they have provided the most inclusive means of encompassing a collective.

C. Wright Mills argued that the mass media have contributed to the erosion of community.[4] His argument is based upon a view of receptive audiences sitting before television screens and receiving messages, which in turn, reinforce privatism and isolation. In particular, Mills saw the danger of passive participation – experiencing the external world via the mass media – as the erosion of man's power to control his destiny. Since members of the audience do not interact but react, communication is one-way.

According to Mills, the mass media do more than inform: they present images of groups and persons, and, in the process, give men personalities. Pseudo-events are fed to us daily, and, through manipulation, particular kinds of situation are controlled, destroyed, changed, or emphasized. The media aggravate conditions in the wider consumer society by encouraging us to take rather than give.

Mills's view undoubtedly has elements of truth, but it may be overstated and it has been modified by subsequent research. The mythical television audience may not be quietly sitting back watching, but may be simultaneously engrossed in other activities or more actively responding. People have always been subject to persuasion, if not from the mass media, from churches and governments, or, more effectively, from the smaller unit of the family. Most of us are quite skilled in techniques of 'ignoring'. Furthermore, it may be said that, as we become more accustomed to our technological inventions, we may develop means of actually talking back and of converting our passive responses into active channels of communication. In fact, the mass media have been heralded by some as the precursors of a new era in international community. We know now about events throughout the entire world in a matter of minutes; wars are fought on the evening news reports while we eat dinner; strange and distant cities are but a switch away. As a result, the globe has become a 'media community' and provides some aspects of a common culture. According to Peter Schrag:

The media – television, radio and records – are creating communities where none existed before. Media are creating bonds of style, age and interest that transcend the particularities of the locality and background. The surface manifestations of a style may themselves satisfy the longing for place and identity, providing alternatives for neighbourhoods, rituals, and traditions that no longer exist.[5]

THE POTENTIAL OF MASS COMMUNICATIONS

It is clear that the receiver does not accept 'pure' messages, but constantly modifies what he receives by factors within his social environment. In addition to his personal distortions and perceptions, there are wider constraints within the social system, such as the expectations of others, which affect the content and delivery of messages. It is not irrational to assume that members of a community select from the media those elements which reinforce their existing beliefs and values. The media may help members to define the boundaries and types of agreed-upon commonalities by reflecting the entire range of social alternatives. In fact, mass communications could become a mediating force between different groups and ideas.

Nor is it so far-fetched to assume that the mass media and other forms of technologically sophisticated communication devices may lead the way to establishing new forms of community in the future. It may upset some to recognize that already many media personalities – commentators, dramatic actors, or newspaper journalists – have a reality for some members of the audience exceeding that of real neighbours or other human contacts. Whenever a 'soap opera' (daytime serial) character, for example, is faced with a traumatic experience, television and radio personnel are barraged with viewer complaints. To many this phenomenon is the archetype of inauthentic social relations, but it need not remain artificial. Television and radio could also provide exciting possibilities for personal contact. The best of children's programmes, 'Blue Peter', for example, constantly urge the child's participation in sponsored events – in the form of letters, pictures, and other feedback communications. The British Broadcasting Corporation provides listeners with the equivalent of 'letters to the editor' columns, long recognized as important channels for personal expression. Educational TV programmes working in conjunction with group participation in discussions and assignments provide a workable conception of receiver participation. Each of these developments stimulates some individual participation, but is it not possible to build *communal* means of participation also? For example, could not a type of student community emerge from the television courses and group discussions that come from the media (e.g. the Open University in Great Britain)?

SOCIAL NETWORKS – AN EXPLANATION

> Men live in a community in virtue of the things which they have in common; and communication is the way in which they come to possess things in common.
>
> *John Dewey*[6]

A social network is a visual picture of the ways in which people surround themselves with others within a personal world or field. The concept of network is borrowed from communications theory. It implies that within a given space one point can be linked with other points, some of which (but not necessarily all) are linked to each other.

Let us imagine a person and his family located at point A, with friends at points B, C, and D. Friends B and D know each other, but neither B nor D knows C, although all know A. In fact, one person may refer to friends B and D in conversation with C and vice versa. The network of contact includes all the significant persons (those whom person A considers important for whatever reasons) even if they should exist in different communities, in many social contexts, and even in widely separated locations.

I have been interested in the concept of social networks since reading a study of twenty ordinary families in London described by Elizabeth Bott in 1957 in her important book *Family and Social Network*. Bott suggested that 'the immediate social environment of an urban family consists of a network rather than an organized group'. She defined a network as a 'social configuration in which some, but not all, of the component external units maintain relationships with one another'.[7] Bott's primary interest was the relationship between conjugal roles and the wider social environment, which she maintains is critical to an understanding of all groups. In the revised edition of *Family and Social Network* she writes:

My aim was (and still is) to understand how the functioning of a group is affected not only by its relationship with the people and organizations of its environment, but also by the relationships among these people and organizations.[8]

If we visualize social relations as clusters of social networks rather than formally bounded groups, an analysis of individual networks may yield significant understandings about the dynamics of interaction. Mitchell and other associates at Manchester have suggested the following characteristics of networks for scrutiny:

1. *Anchorage* – This is usually the person being studied or groups of persons under observation.
2. *Reachability* – The steps between the anchor and the other persons within the network.
3. *Density* – This refers to the degree of connectedness or closeness of contacts.
4. *Range* – How wide are the number of contacts: Does the person know many or few other persons?
5. *Content* – Possibilities here include kinship ties, economic assistance, friendship ties.
6. *Directedness* – Are the links mutual or non-reciprocal?
7. *Durability* – Does the network have different characteristics at different stages of life?
8. *Intensity* – How close are the individual links?
9. *Frequency* – Do the links interact together regularly and frequently?[9]

Could we go further and examine the intersection of many personal social networks; the contact points between different individuals; to see if this might become the incubator of some forms of community? For example, Bott's list of variables which should be studied to determine network density and conjugal segregation, is also a list of critical elements in any community analysis. These include: occupation, geographical mobility, social mobility, ecological factors, subculture and ethnic group, education, phase of individual and family development, various reference groups based on the above factors.[10] Because of increased mobility and cultural transformations in contemporary society, social networks may constitute the dominant social arrangements for individuals, In so doing, they may also constitute a social structure which could be considered a form of community by relating the individual to a public or collectivity.

If these concepts appear amorphous, we need only examine critically our own social experiences. Many of us, in fact, maintain social contacts in a wide variety of contexts: we are loath to identify ourselves as permanent members of a fixed group on the basis of any single set of circumstances. Nor do we restrict our social experiences to kin or neighbours or colleagues, but range widely among many types of association. Yet, we do not consider ourselves without roots or isolated; we can identify some pattern and relationships between our contacts, and we recognize some similarities in social identities. In other words, Bott's conception of social network rings true because the very openness of structure, the variability of elements, and the fluidity of form corresponds to what we experience in everyday life.

One way to identify and locate networks is by an analysis of communication channels. By measuring the flow of communications between points, we are able to diagram and quantify many aspects of interaction. But many questions remain that are pertinent to understanding the juxtaposition of networks. For example, what factors lead persons to enter into another's social world? When do individuals choose to belong together or identify with others? What factors make it possible for individuals to come together and find social satisfactions in a wider connection than with isolated individuals or family? I suggest that when individuals have an opportunity to express themselves emotionally and rationally; when the individual is encouraged to mediate between conflicting role demands; and when he recognizes a mutuality of interest and concern with others; his network provides the structure for communal development.

Bott has argued that the concept of social network is not new. Members of an educated elite, for example, share a common network in spite of distance or nationality. Similarly, military officers, business executives, and other 'sophisticated' types are able to expand their social worlds beyond geographical borders into a social network transcending many normal boundaries. Historically there have always been groups that have done this: in churches, business, education (the old-boy network). The social circle has provided writers with abundant materials for many years, representing a small intimate group which could be thought of as a unit or group cornerstone of the communal structure.

The significance of social-network analysis is that it may help us understand how men have responded to conditions of modern life to meet their social needs.

SOCIAL NETWORKS IN AN URBAN UNIVERSITY

Following Bott's example, I was curious to see if social networks could provide tracks that might lead to the discovery of urban communal structures. I attempted to map out the social networks of 52 students living at home and in flats who attended Chelsea College of Technology in central London.[11]

After two intensive interviews, each student was asked to record all contacts for a two-week period and to explain the importance of the people with whom he had dealings. In some instances, I visited the students' homes to meet people who they had suggested were central in their social world.

Within the sample, I found many variations and differences between students regarding the range of contacts, and the number and depth of relationships. Yet there were also significant similarities and forms that revealed patterns in social organizations that could conceivably become communal structures.

The most difficult research problem in determining the amount of cohesion among networks – and by this is meant in evaluating how close-knit or loose-knit was the student's network or how many of the links were connected with each other – was the matter of family. Naturally, the student living at home has more contact with his family than the student living away; although the amount of contact revealed nothing about the strength of feelings between the student and his family or the importance of the ties. For this reason, it became necessary for the student himself to evaluate the importance of home social life, and this subjective qualitative evaluation was used as the basis for determining whether or not the student was socially close to or distant from his kin.

Another difficulty was the problem of measuring depth. For the student 'going steady' or engaged, it sometimes became necessary to restrict the number of other contacts in order to find time to be with the 'special' person. In some cases, the student was able to maintain a balance between his major personal interest and frequent interaction with others. However, other sacrificed the range of associates for more penetrating relationships with one or two others. The variation in range and depth no doubt reflected personality differences (i.e. the extrovert would tend to extend his range, the introvert restrict his) but very important 'structural' and sociological factors affected these characteristics of social networks also.

NETWORKS AND ROLE ORIENTATIONS

The most striking influence upon the student's social network was his definition of the student's role. For example, some students adopted a collegiate orientation toward student life. By this is meant that college life, both academically and socially, was their main interest. As a result, almost all friends and acquaintances were centred upon the college and these contacts, in turn, knew each other. Because the 'collegiate' (by this I mean a student who views his college life as the centre of all social, intellectual, and personal activities) participated in many college activities, generally lived with other students, and in cases of 'going steady' went with a girl or boy from the college, his or her social network was close-knit and wide-ranging. This contrasted clearly with the student who viewed his student role as vocational training. He attended the college to prepare himself for a specific field, and to obtain training for his career. As a result, this student was not particularly interested in college activities because they disturbed his prime concern with advanced training. His friends were restricted to department workmates at the college, and, at home, to his family or a few flatmates. The vocationally oriented student frequently lived in two distinct social worlds – the college and outside college.

Another type of social network that was affected by the student's orientation towards his role was that of the academic student. In this instance, the student was seriously concerned with academic work, making friends from a variety of spheres, and was comfortable in a non-personal situation because he enjoyed ideas and things. His social network could be wide-ranging or restricted. The fourth student orientation was that of the nonconforming individual, seeking his own identity from many experiences, and creating a loose-knit, wide-ranging network; sometimes building intense relationships with one person for a brief time, but breaking off to wander on to others.

SOCIAL NETWORK AND COMMUNITY

Two interesting conclusions about social networks were related directly to contemporary community. First, it was not accomodation or locality or any other geographical factors that played the most significant part in the organization of the student's social structure, but his orientation towards the student role. This provided the core of commonness or a student culture that became the framework for building social networks.

Second, contrary to the popular view, there was actually a form of student community at Chelsea. It was geographically dispersed, constantly changing, and hard to separate from the other collectivities that existed in this situation: the college as an educational institution and Chelsea as an operating organization. But the students were not isolated individuals: they shared a common orientation towards an important part of their lives (college); followed common mores and norms; agreed upon many values and goals: had opportunity for personal communication with each other; and in general, were able to build together a social structure that could be identified as communal.

The identification of the Chelsea student community by means of social network analysis suggests that communities do, in fact, exist in urban contexts, within institutional boundaries, and amid many other social collectivities. The lack of boundaries made one suspect conditions of anomie, but the everyday lives of many students did not support this conclusion. In this densely packed social environment, through a network created to communicate personally meaningful and important messages, the students shared their commonness. The network indicated a structure that was not distinct from the rest of the environment, but patterned and organized parts of the social experience into a form of community.

In modern societies it may be at the intersection of several personal networks that persons have an opportunity to develop social structures that meet some, if not all, of the requirements of a community. Here, the person may express himself emotionally and intellectually; mediate between conflicting role demands; recognize a wider, public sector in his life. This new form of community would deal with the demand of modern life for choice and mobility, and be one way to create social collectives based upon personal values.

COMMENTS ON SOCIAL NETWORK RESEARCH

As the example illustrates, most of the research on social networks has been exploratory and experimental. We have not yet refined the concepts precisely enough to permit wide-scale investigation, nor have we developed techniques by which we can adequately trace the many diverse elements within a network.

The work of researchers at Manchester University is particularly relevant to these concerns.[12] J. Clyde Mitchell's nine criteria for the classification of social networks have been described.

Another important source of information related to network analysis is to be found in the sociometric studies that reveal the patterns of social choices among individuals. Studies revealing the direction and amounts of communication between persons are also important.

However, there are serious questions still outstanding. For example, we do not understand how the network operates to hold persons together. Our pictures are of different personal social worlds that combine one person and his peculiar arrangements. Although each network must reflect initially the personal characteristics of the individual, it seems possible that social patterns are also reflected, since so many aspects of the individual's world are determined by social factors, e.g. social class, the stage of his life-cycle, and the overall social milieux in which he lives, but there are few empirical sudies to verify this.[13]

We need to know a great deal more about the range of contacts among people not geographically contiguous. For example,[14] we know that the average town-dweller does not depend upon neighbourhood or work contacts alone. As noted in the discussion of the family, research demonstrates also that he maintains contact with his kin, visiting relatives frequently. In spite of mobility there are many long-standing friendships that play a significant role in the person's life. From these, the town-dweller builds a social world about him made up of a variety of contacts from many different sources. Some of these contacts know each other: workmates, for example, or family members interact among themselves and with him. His wife and children share many of these social contacts, but a few remain private linkages with only the individual. In short, we need to trace private and shared networks more carefully.

The concept of social networks is not confined to a search for localized communities. Members of the educated elite, for example, share a common network in spite of distance or nationality. Similarly, military officers, business executives, and others are able to expand private social worlds beyond the communal borders into a social network that transcends ordinary boundaries of nationality, culture, or profession. Historically, there have always been groups who have done this: in churches, business, or education. This is what is popularly recognized as the 'old boy network' and visibly witnessed by the school-tie. It is also the basis for identification by means of a special language – the regional accent, the professional jargon, the contemporary slang – which is transmitted along social networks in many different social settings.

Because of increased mobility and communications, the intersections of several personal networks are increasingly fluid, mixed, and not clearly defined. But if the person can express himself emotionally and intellectually in a network mediating between conflicting role demands; recognize a wider, public sector in his life; and respond to social demands selectively, he has, in fact, developed with others a form of community.

At the present stage, social network analysis remains an exciting and stimulating possible means of understanding human relationships in situations where the usual social structures are not observed and contacts appear scattered and diffused. Many will dismiss the concept of contacts located in a wide social network as vague, impossible to verify, and confusing. Yet the concept comes closer to our individual understandings of our private social worlds than the others described. With computer assistance, growing social-scientific sophistication, better observational tools, and more penetrating theoretical understandings, it may yet be possible to find ways of mapping social networks to see if they do form the foundations of communities. They certainly provide one of our best clues to locating modern community, although admittedly we have much to investigate.

11 And so, where are we?

It is a question of identity
and whether I am really I,
and whether you are you,
Can this be a community
composed of the most peculiar I
and more peculiar you?
Kevin Maguire[1]

Our discussion has ranged across many areas, possible creating more questions than it has answered. Our task is now briefly to retrace our steps and see where we have moved in our search for modern forms of community.

In the discussion we have frequently used the terms 'structure' and 'form'. The traditional social-scientific approach has been to study given societies, noting the social structures that exist, to describe these, and then explain how they function to keep the entire social system operating.[2] In such an approach, communities are located within the system, and the analyst proceeds to determine how these communities meet social needs. Our approach is somewhat different. We have assumed, as a starting-point, that men do not live alone, taking as given the biological, economic, political, and psychological reasons for this. Then we have asked, if not alone – how together? Surveying the answers revealed that there were as many and varied types of social forms as there are men and societies. From among these, we selected one – community – by starting with the experiences of participants and gradually moving to the structures that have evolved.

The advantages of the 'search and see' approach is that we are not restricted by rigid prescriptions, treading over the same old research paths. We do not have to find community in the expected places: e.g.

among the poor or in a particular administrative locality. It follows, also, that we do not locate personal alienation and conditions of anomie in many familiar settings, but can question many commonly held presuppositions about living arrangements in modern societies. In short, our imaginations are freer, our eyes more wide-ranging, and our searching more diverse.

The disadvantages of this approach are also evident. In particular, there is the charge of vagueness. The communities we locate are not clearly bounded and are mixed with many other social forms. They do not seem precise or definite because they are not anchored by geography, life-styles, or isolation. They are unfamiliar and strange.

Yet, my own experience of reality (and I think that of many others) suggests that this view of social organization comes close to the experience of living in technologically advanced, urban societies. The people with whom I associate and the patterns of my own life do not fit neatly into any categories, and certainly not that of a traditional community. I interact in many congruent, overlapping, and changing social forms at the same time. My relationships with other associates in many different social structures are based upon a variety of roles, and the social bonds that tie me to different associations are complex, numerous, and confused.

Another difficulty concerning the communal forms that we locate by 'wandering' is that they have little of the historical stability of earlier communities. They seem ephemeral, constantly changing, and so temporary as to appear insignificant. Once again, in a critical review of my own experience, I see that my communities are not as permanent as those of my parents. I am not at all certain that my community of today will be the same as that of next year, and I am almost certain that the community of my children will be different from mine in the future.

SOCIOLOGICAL APPROACHES

> . . . the imaginations which people have of one another are the solid facts of society. . . .
>
> *Charles Cooley*[3]

As a study based upon empirical evidence, sociology must relate to the reality we experience in everyday life. But this is not easy in the case of rapidly changing social forms. Our research tools and our intellectual concepts are all geared to a study of fixed social matter, just as the physicists' orientation was to a universe held together by uniform forces of nature. The sociological problems are even greater. Our techniques are based upon: (1) observation – but most of our intellectual equipment produces still-life pictures rather than moving scenes, (2) asking questions of subjects – but our subjects interpret our words so differently that, when we have recorded it all, no one is really too sure what the replies mean, or (3) measurement – but we have not been very successful in evaluating qualitative variables that play such a significant part in the ordering of social priorities.

C. Wright Mills complained that, in an effort to avoid criticism, we have adopted trite questions for research – they mean little but our techniques are adequate.[4] Or we have substituted political rhetoric about the coming revolution which will abolish all existing social structures, substituting instead direct personal relationships. The absurdity of this view – millions of men acting randomly without any patterns of organization, purpose, or rules – is as ridiculous as the opposite view: that most of life is planned, orderly, and coherent. Specifically, in terms of community, we have defined the term so narrowly on the basis of a comparatively few anthropological studies and habitual labels adopted by administrative units for convenience, that we have convinced ourselves that community does not exist.

Sociologists, have become too conservative, too concerned with what people say society is and where it is, instead of saying: 'Let's see where it might be and what might be relevant to peoples' lives.' We cannot conclude anything unless we go out and see what is; and we cannot find out what is unless we take a few risks in looking!

Let us agree that if we mean by community the traditional association of the past, community does not exist in many urban situations and it is likely that it will not exist in the future. But to leap from this observation to the conclusion than men live alone, or in meaningless social aggregates, is not only unrealistic, but also indicative of a kind of sociological blindness. In the preceeding pages we have attempted in a modest and clumsy way to see if some forms of communal association can be found if the term is interpreted in a more comprehensive manner. I think that we have found some evidence that communities do exist.

But before going further, it must be repeated that, in three-quarters of the globe, the type of community established is that of the traditional community of place. Commonality continues to develop from a shared culture, occupation, and religion, and from isolation. Recognizing this, serious observers stress the importance of giving aid to these communities so that they may retain their individuality, strength and importance. Nor is an interest in modern forms of community a rejection of this view. It is, rather, an attempt to discuss the question in a different context – that of technologically advanced urbanized societies. Under these conditions, I suggest that communities are divorced from place, that cultural differentiation has been reduced, and that the pervading ethos of change and movement prevents the formation of permanent associations.

We are now able to discuss four forms of community as illustrative of the collectives that can be located in modern societies. They are:

1. certain types of social network
2. synthetic communities based upon approximations of natural or traditional communities of place and culture
3. hybrids composed of institutions or organizations that adopt essential communal characteristics
4. the intense, short-lived temporary community

Let us look at each of these briefly.

SOCIAL NETWORKS

The concept of social network is basically a view of community that begins with individuals, examines the various components of the person's social world, and attempts to find patterns of linkage or connection between components. Each person develops a unique and personal network reflecting the sum total of his private choices and his own social characteristics. Because many of us are affected by the same social factors, e.g. class, occupation, age, or culture, it is likely that there are many overlaps between social networks among different groups. At these intersections, or the linking points between different persons, one can diagram a community structure.

At the present time this concept has been only vaguely defined and researched, so our discussion may appear more theoretical than realistic. Although a great deal of study and clarification is needed, the process of locating persons in a social field in which network links overlap and touch, is a provocative attempt to explain those situations in which persons cannot be identified by formal groupings or definite organizational structures.

SYNTHETIC COMMUNITIES

A synthetic community is an attempt to build and develop a community consciously and deliberately. Some writers maintain that this is impossible, as Greeley writes:

> Community can't be rushed or sought directly and self-consciously . . . Community is neither a goal nor a means. It is, rather, a side effect resulting from continued interaction between human beings. It enriches and facilitates more interaction but it must stem from and be rooted in interaction. Men must have something to do together before they can become a community, and those who pursue community as an end in itself will be as disappointed as those who pursue happiness as an end in itself.[5]

In this, Greeley reminds us that simply placing people side by side is no guarantee that they will share anything in common. This is particularly true when people move from one social context to another in the course of a single day. It also explains why many of the ambitious town-planning programmes have not borne communal fruit. As the study of Levittown revealed, it may be in defining how we are different from our neighbours – in the conflict over what is to be called community as well as what is shared in common – that genuine communities develop.

However, before we dismiss the idea of synthetic communities as unworkable, we must carefully examine the advantages of such social engineering. Some argue that only if society sustains community by a deliberate social intent, careful planning, and direction can communities flourish and grow.

Many of our important life-concepts are, in fact, synthetic devices by which we can control our destiny and find a place for ourselves within the universe, for men require forms and patterns to remove uncertainty. If community can provide a satisfying and meaningful context in which man may order many of his social relationships, stimulating communal development by artificial means is worth while. Furthermore, it may be possible to use technological devices to assist creating synthetic communities along unexplored and imaginative lines.

HYBRIDS

Some institutions and organizations have become more community-like. They have adopted many of the characteristics of a community, combining them with other goals. There is a danger that such combinations will become inauthentic, using the communal forms to resolve the usual difficulties found in large-scale operations: impersonality, individual isolation, inadequate kinds of communication, or, most importantly, loss of commitment on the part of participants. By convincing others that the social arrangements are communal, leaders may simply attempt to soften the image of a ruthless, efficient, and inhuman bureaucracy, and use community as a social mask.

However, there are examples of hybrid communities that are more successful at the merger. One example is the development of professional communities. For the individual devoted to a professional career, it is possible to build his occupational life at the heart of a host of related activities that extend into the personal sphere. These activities range from social clubs to residential facilities. Partly this is brought about by the long period of training and apprenticeship that the professional undergoes prior to achieving his status. Even after the original preparation, the individual must continue to study and keep up with professional matters, so that structures to communicate information are established and other structures – to police members and enforce standards, to assist in recruitement, and to speak for the interests of the profession – are initiated.

Religious groups and educational institutions, particularly boarding schools or universities, in some instances, consciously try to become communities. Many never achieve full communal status, but some do, in fact, become more like a community than an institution. This is also true for some organizations when personal and collective goals become blurred.

TEMPORARY, INTIMATE COMMUNITIES

The intense, short-lived community is one established for a brief period – a weekend, a week, or a few months. Members interact intensely and deeply throughout this period, becoming almost completely emotionally involved. The sheer intensity of this interaction means that such a community could not be sustained for long periods of time because members would have to forgo all other concerns in order to devote themselves totally to their communal interests. Once the community achieves some permanence, the charisma and emotional intensity gradually become routinized and controlled. When this occurs, the community is transformed into a different type of association, and members who originally joined to fulfil personal and emotional needs for intense association often become dissatisfied and leave.

Examples of short-lived communities are growing in modern society for many reasons. Mobility makes it possible for people today to meet together in different contexts for brief periods, and then return to normal life activities. Second, the demands of specialization in life activities has meant that only by planning to be part of a totally engrossing activity for a brief period can the individual be free to invest the emotional capital required in some of these attempts. Third, this form of community – brief, intense and complete – meets the needs of those who seek community according to private interest and tastes.

Communes often form such short-lived communities. Although communes generally set out as long-term associations, they are usually forced to disband or transform themselves because of the very emotional tensions that led to their formation originally. At times, residential conferences or absorbing work projects that isolate participants from others become brief communal experiences. This is not to say that all of these automatically become communities. The requirements for structure, for public concern, and for integration of member roles must still be met. Many intense associations remain small groups. But those which extend beyond the group stage, may, in fact, become temporary communities.

COMMUNITY IN MODERN CONTEXTS – A SUMMARY

Certain essentials are required in any community: a 'core of commonness' or communality that includes a collective perspective, agreed-upon definitions, and some agreement about values. Communities are unique social collectives because they provide a context for personal integration. Here the individual adopts some social priorities in order to reformulate conflicting life-styles (or protect himself against them). The adjective 'personal' limits the integrative function of community, for it is clear that communities actively compete with each other or are in direct conflict with both smaller and larger aggregates. (Although from this diversity a wider social integration based upon dependence, toleration, and mobility may develop). Members of a community are committed to the community to the extent of identifying directly or indirectly with the whole, and by having shared rather than functional social bonds with others.

The reasons why there is a renewed interest in community are many. Among them has been the desire to find an antidote to excessive individualism, but the wish to reduce atomization usually leads to a romanticized view of togetherness, and the reality of community as a social structure, a way of ordering social relationships with both positive and negative affects, is forgotten. Another source of interest can be traced to the destruction of social myths. For example, the image of 'good' communities is implicit in the view of the pure countryside and the evil city. There is a danger in destroying myths. As pointed out earlier, Schon argues that we must believe in stability in order to reduce the uncertainty of change. Traditionally, man has used ritual as a technique for doing this, but according to Douglas:

> One of the gravest problems of our day is the lack of commitment to common symbols. If this were all, there would be little to say. If it were merely a matter of our fragmentation into small groups, each committed to its proper symbolic forms, the case would be simple to understand. But more mysterious is a wide-spread explicit rejection of rituals as such. Ritual is become a bad word signifying empty conformity. We are witnessing a revolt against formalism, even against form.[6]

Her explanation in terms of group – the experience of a bonded social unit and grid, the rules that relate one person to another on an ego-centred basis – is useful, for the two are found in the context of community as outlined above.

Looking at community critically makes the concept far less grandiose: few people get excited about a social form. Yet for those interested in restructuring society realistically, such an understanding is more practical.

CONCLUSION

What can we conclude at the end of our exploring? If anything, it is simply that the conditions of modern life require a constant re-appraisal and re-analysis of all our conceptual tools. We cannot face modern reality with old ideas because they no longer apply. If we redefine our social forms, using as guidelines the reality about us that can be empirically documented through social research, then we may yet find viable, meaningful, and important social structures that have been created in response to new human needs and values.

And, it goes without saying, as we redefine our social arrangements, we redefine ourselves. To undertake such activity in a deliberate, thoughtful, and humane attempt to live together peacefully must be our goal.

Postscript A new function for communities – humanizing systems

The great frontier today is the exploration of the human potential, man's seemingly limitless ability to adapt, to grow, to invent his own destiny. There is much to learn; but we already know this: the future need not happen to us; we can make it happen.

R. Farson[1]

Historically, communities have provided the means by which men have been able to live together. Originally they helped men to obtain economic sustenance, protection against enemies, and assistance in growth, as required by every new-born human being. Gradually, communities became the social expression of common beliefs, values, and meanings, not only providing man with the physical resources for survival, but the intellectual, moral, and social values to give purpose to that survival. To some extent all communities continue to do this today.

But modern communities may have a further purpose. New communities, changed dramatically in form from old villages, exist within huge systems that encompass organizations, institutions, groups, individuals, and other communities in overall patterns of action. The control and direction of such systems is presently left to men specialized in one particular aspect of life and expert in particular processes of the overall composite. As a result, the only agreed-upon criterion for evaluating systems operations has been efficiency.[2]

What is required is a context for integrating these systems, a social structure in which the goals and objectives of efficient operations are discussed and in which men can commit themselves to the moral uses of systems. Such a context is community. Here groups of individuals can do what no individual can do alone: here, we can find the political power, social commitment, vital interest and concern, and the human resources, to control and change our destiny.

Our view is that communal man is able to bring into focus those issues which have escaped the attention of specialists: he can insist through the social structures of community that additional factors enter debate, creating a platform for raising new terms and suggesting viable alternatives to standardized systems and programmes.

Said simply, the potential of community – both as a way of thinking and as a social form – is to humanize systems. Let me explain: of all the social arrangements available to man in which he can pursue human objectives, community provides the richest context in which he can cooperate with others. Only when man is viewed as a whole being do the disharmonies and discontinuities of life become visible. This does not mean that such an association will be free from conflict or stress: we speak of communities not utopias. Nor does it mean that community provides a structural solution to the critical problems of human life: communities only offer a multidimensional environment in which to examine these issues.

To humanize systems – bringing men back to the centre of existence – will not, in itself, make the world a better place to live in. For individuals, like the communities they develop as the social expressions of shared values and beliefs, are from the perfect. All that can be said in favour of a *human system* is that the debates and discussions will at least be concerned with human values rather than with technological and synthetic ends. In short, by reintroducing moral considerations in all areas, the humanization of systems becomes, in fact, the province of community.

Sometimes, to be sure, one wonders if human concerns are more intelligent or humane than those mechanically devised! But if our choice is to be human or not or, perhaps more accurately, to accept the responsibility for being human or not, I, for one, prefer the former. But it must be remembered that, historically, most communities have been more effective in obstructing, confusing, and prohibiting larger systems from operating than in creating conditions for positive change. And it is also true that most people still regard community as a stable, unchanging, and rigid social form of little value in changing or redirecting powerful systems. The unique characteristic of community is that members can express common concern over values, beliefs, and goals, thereby becoming a potential force to stimulate change. According to David Minar and Scott Greer:[3]

> . . . community is both empirically descriptive of a social structure and normatively toned. It refers both to the unit of society as it is and to the aspects of the unit that are valued if they exist, desired in their absence. Community is indivisible from humane actions, purposes and values. It expresses our vague yearnings for a commonality of desire, a communion with those around us, an extension of bonds of kin and friend to all those who share a common fate with us.

BY WAY OF ENDING . . .

> Effective action depends not on finding the right answers, but discovering paths – or to use the jargon, tracks for continuous adjustment to changing, not to say, clashing conditions. 'Only connect' – E. M. Forster's famous motto – is in fact, the first commandment of the new gospel.
>
> *Joseph Kraft*[4]

We seldom discover anything that it is genuinely new and different. Rather, creativity is the process of rearranging old ideas to develop new perspectives and reveal old problems in different lights. The concept of community is as old as civilization. However, the forms of community have radically altered in many turbulent environments. Our search for new forms is an attempt to rearrange our ideas about social structures in order to find those ways in which modern men have expressed their commonality. For it is only in so doing that we can bring men back into the centre of the many complex systems that dominate our lives. In so doing, we may yet regain the pride and joyousness of being human, and of sharing with others.

General bibliography

The following are general works of interest to a reader who wishes to continue the study of communities. Each represents a significant contribution to our understanding of modern communities and has been incorporated into the ideas presented in this discussion.

ARENSBERG, C. AND KIMBALL, S. 1965 *Culture and community*. New York: Harcourt Brace and World. The authors view community as a sample to study complex cultures and societies, or 'a master institution or master social system; a key to society; and a model, indeed perhaps the most important model, of culture'. The link between society and culture is community, and current community studies represent a method of developing both concepts and programmes.

COX, H. 1965 *The secular city*. New York: Macmillan; Harmondsworth: Penguin. Although Cox is primarily concerned with religion in modern societies, his reflections upon the effects of urbanization in social relations are an important contribution to an understanding of contemporary communities.

ETZIONI, A. 1968 *A theory of societal and political processes: the active society*. New York: The Free Press; London: Collier-Macmillan. Etzioni deals with large-scale communities, such as nation-states, in most of the discussion. He provides a comprehensive assessment of the development of societies, and an indispensable reference to significant social literature on the topic.

FRANKENBERG, R. 1966 *Communities in Britain: social life in town and country*. Harmondsworth: Penguin. Frankenberg develops a continuum upon which he compares communities ranging from rural hamlets to urban areas. He suggests useful criteria for comparing different communities along sociological themes, including one adopted in this discussion: social network analysis.

KÖNIG, R. 1968 *The community*. E. FITZGERALD (trans.) London: Routledge and Kegan Paul. König traces the development of the concept 'community' from its Germanic roots, explains how it was adopted by French intellectuals, and presents the basis for considering community as an empirical reality. It is a solid theoretical foundation upon which further inquiry can be based.

MINAR, D. AND GREER, S. 1969 *The concept of community*. Chicago: Aldine; London: Butterworth. This is a book or readings, with brief but provocative interpretations. Selections range from classical social science to contemporary literature and make up an impressive collection of original sources.

NISBET, R. 1962 *Community and power*. New York: Oxford University Press; 1967 *The sociological tradition*. London: Heinemann. Both of these deal extensively with the development of community as a sociological concept and as a political concept. Nisbet provides the theoretical understandings which explain why community has remained a significant idea throughout history.

REDFIELD, R. 1955 *Little community: comparative studies of cultures and civilizations*. Chicago: University of Chicago Press. This is a classic statement of the anthropological approach to the study of small communities.

STEIN, M. 1960 *The eclipse of community*. New York: Harper and Row. Stein provides an interpretation of American community studies, as well as the foundations for an interdisciplinary approach to community studies.

WARREN, R. L. 1966 *Perspectives on the American community*. Chicago: Rand-McNally. This is an inclusive list of readings, both modern and classical, on community in America. Section One: 'Basic approaches to the community' is a particularly useful orientation towards the literature.

Notes

Preface

1. PEIRCE, C. S. 1868 Some consequences of four incapacities. *Journal of Speculative Philosophy.* Reprinted in: R. J. WILSON (ed.) 1968. *In quest of community.* New York: John Wiley.

Chapter 1

1. ARDREY, R. 1967 *The territorial imperative,* p. 111. London: Collins.
2. Confusion over the use of the term 'community' may be seen in a collection of more than ninety definitions by G. HILLERY: Villages, cities, and total institutions. *American Sociological Review* Vol. 28, 1964. A practical illustration of the difficulties in applying community was the reception given to the Youth Service Development Council's Report *Youth and community work in the 70's.* According to BERNARD DAVIS, 'Nothing in the document seems to have caused greater confusion than its frequent references to "community and community work".' *New Society* 19 March 1970.
3. KAPLAN, A. 1964 *The conduct of inquiry.* San Francisco: Chandler. He writes: 'Openness of meaning is fundamentally a consequence of the fact that there are no terminal contexts of inquiry' (p. 70). Kaplan argues that creativity requires a tolerance for ambiguity.
4. ETZIONI, A. 1967 *The active society: a theory of societal and political processes,* p. 2. New York: The Free Press; London: Collier-Macmillan.
5. NISBET, R. 1966 *The sociological tradition,* p. 47. London: Heinemann.
6. DURKHEIM, E. *The division of labour in society.* G. SIMPSON (trans.) Glencoe: The Free Press, 1947; London: Collier-Macmillan. This represents the classical sociological discussion of changes brought about in industrial societies. Many of these ideas are taken from the writings of Frederick Tönnies. See: *Gemeinschaft and Gesellschaft.* G. LOOMIS (trans.) New York: The American Book Company, 1940. For a general discussion of the differences in sociological approaches see: P. BERGER 1963 *Invitation to sociology: a humanistic perspective.* Harmondsworth: Penguin.

7. Marx is confusing to read on this subject because he looks with disdain upon communities of place (which he regards as rural holdovers) but welcomes the psychological community of common interests. He writes: 'Only in community with others has each individual the means of cultivating his gifts in all directions. In the real community the individuals obtain their freedom in and through their associations.' K. MARX: The German ideology, in T. BOTTOMORE and M. RUBEL (eds.), *Selected writings in sociology and social philosophy*. Harmondsworth; Penguin, 1963.
8. WEBER, M. *From Max Weber*. H. GERTH and C. W. MILLS (eds.). London: Routledge 1948.
9. BENNIS, W. and SLATER, P. 1968 *The temporary society*. New York: Harper and Row.
10. MOYNIHAN, D. O. Eliteland. *Psychology Today* September 1970, p. 68. Writing as an adviser to the President of the United States, Moynihan is concerned with the American situation. He argues that social scientists have assumed a 'priestly role' and feels that only by recognizing the areas of inadequacy and re-examining social science with a critical view, can these be of any value in guiding political decisions.
11. DURKHEIM, E. *The rules of sociological method*. K. WOLFF (ed.). London: Collier-Macmillan, 1950. Durkheim explained social facts as follows: 'Here then is a category of facts with very distinctive characteristics: it consists of ways of acting, thinking and feeling, external to the individual, and endowed with a power of coercion, by reason of which they control him. These ways of thinking could not be confused with biological phenomena, since they consist of representations and of actions, nor with psychological phenomena, which exist only in the individual's consciousness and through it. They constitute a new variety of phenomena: and it is to them exclusively that the term social ought to be applied. These ways of thinking and acting therefore constitute the proper domain of sociology.'
12. MILLS, C. W. 1959 *The sociological imagination*. New York: The Free Press, p. 3. Harmondsworth: Penguin, p. 19.
13. MICHAEL, D. N. 1968 *The unprepared society*, p. 14. New York: Basic Books.
14. Moynihan's point is that for most of the world (excepting homogeneous populations) ethnicity persists and is 'extraordinarily important, if not central to the problem'. It must be noted that his 'conservative approach' is to redirect social scientists from interest in class to ethnic differentials, and represents the continuity of the Durkheimian heritage.
15. GOULDNER, A. 1970 *The coming crisis of Western sociology* London: Heinemann, 1971. Also: Anti-minotaur: the myth of value-free sociology. *Social Problems* Winter 1962. Similar arguments are found in: T. S. SIMEY 1968 *Social science and social purpose*. London: Constable. It is also summarized succinctly in these words: 'To the extent that a sociological theory addresses itself directly to the notion that man is conscious of the world he lives in, is aware of the meanings and

intentions of his actions, to the extent of this, the theory presents a subjective point of view.' C. S. FENTON The myth of subjectivism as a special method in sociology. *The Sociological Review* vol. 16:3 November 1968. The discussion presented in the personal introduction is part of Mills's admonition to perceive of sociology as the fusion of personal biography and social issues.

16. The evidence that some men lead satisfying or sustaining lives must be the reality of functioning systems. One could cite the various surveys which attempt to measure different types of satisfaction, or refer to studies which cite degrees of well-being. However, if the argument is based on the assumption that we do not have adequate measures of qualitative experiences, or sufficient research based upon investigation of these questions, it seems illogical to cite these as evidence.

Chapter 2

1. STEINBECK, J. Autobiography: making of a New Yorker. *New York Times Magazine* 1 February 1953.
2. CULLEN, P. and CULLEN, G. Paradoxes of mobility. *The Times* (London) 12 July 1968.
3. JONES, M. The untouchables. *The Observer Review* 3 November 1968.
4. MCCLENAHAN, B. A. The communality: the urban substitute for the traditional community *Sociology and social research* vol. XXX, March–April 1946, pp. 264–271.
5. MARTINSEN, F. M. 1970 Family class and community. Chapter Nine in *Family in society*. New York: Dodd, Mead and Company.
6. STRAUSS, A. 1968 *The American city: a sourcebook of urban imagery*, p. 8. London: Allen Lane.
7. MILLS, C. W. The professional ideology of social pathologies. *American Journal of Sociology* vol. 49, 1943.
8. BLYTHE, R. 1969 *Akenfield: a portrait of an English village*. London: Allen Lane; New York: Pantheon. This is an excellent description of rural village life. It should be noted that much of the poverty of the Third World is rural in character. This is supported in American studies. See: A. SHOSTAK and W. GOMBERG 1965. *New perspectives on poverty*. Englewood Cliffs: Prentice-Hall.
9. GIST, N. and FAVA, S. 1964 *Urban society*, p. 88. 5th edition, New York: Thomas Crowell.
10. GREER, S. 1962 *The emerging city*, p. 194. Glencoe: The Free Press.
11. PARK, R. The city. *American Journal of Sociology* 1915. See also: R. PARK and E. BURGESS 1921. *Introduction to the science of sociology*. Chicago: University of Chicago Press.
12. ALEXANDER, C. The city as a mechanism for sustaining human contact. In W. EWALD (ed.) 1967. *Environment for man*, p. 65. Bloomington:

Indiana University Press. See also: H. COX 1968 *On not leaving it to the snake*. London: SCM Press. Cox writes: 'It is probably true that the present erosion of our sense of place has resulted in part from the secularization of our culture with its tendency to divest space of any sacral significance. It has arisen also from high mobility, always accompanied by less reverence for place, and by the technological mentality of our time which allows men to rearrange the material world freely and without undue reference to some presumed inherent significance intrinsic in it' (p. 117). See also: M. STEIN (ed.) 1960 The restoration of a sense of place. *The eclipse of community*. New York: Harper and Row.

13. WIRTH, L. 1964 Urbanism as a way of life. A. REISS (ed.), *On cities and social life*. Chicago, London: University of Chicago Press, p. 190.
14. MEAD, M. 1970 *Culture and commitment*. New York: Doubleday. Paradoxically, many environmentalists believe that by creating communities of place, they can develop an ethic of caring for the physical area, noting how many successful conservation movements have been based on this. William Whyte argues cogently, however, that environmentalists do not succeed when they say no and simply restrict areas, since the problems generally encompass wider sections. To reject without providing realistic alternatives delays and frustrates solutions to environmental problems. W. WHYTE 1970 *The last landscape*. New York: Doubleday.
15. MCLUHAN, M. and FIORE, Q. 1967 *The medium is the message*. New York: Bantam. Also: M. MCLUHAN 1964 *Understanding media*. London: Routledge & Kegan Paul.
16. LEACH, E. Communities. *New society*, 15 May 1969.
17. GRAND, E. Life in an instant village. *Nova* February 1970. Another study of the Span Estate is being conducted by the Sociological Research Unit of University College. See: J. BARR Status village. *New society*, October 1969. It should be noted that these estates have populations of between five and six thousand and cannot be strictly compared to Levittown in terms of size and complexity.
18. GANS, H. 1967 *The Levittowners*. London: Allen Lane. Another useful discussion of suburbia, particularly with regard to the myths surrounding its development is: S. DONALDSON 1969 *The suburban myth*. New York: Columbia University Press. In this, Donaldson incorporates the developments of suburbia in the United States with the Jeffersonian ideal, tracing the disillusionment resulting from failure to the power of this ideal rather than to social reality. Another important contribution is: J. ORR and F. NICHELSON 1970 *The radical suburb: soundings in changing American character*. Philadelphia: Westminster Press. This is a psychological examination of some of the sociological themes regarding suburbia in America. The authors argue that the image of conservative, middle-class suburban attitudes does not take into account a new consciousness which has been developed within the last five years.
19. Op. cit. Gans, p. 408. See also: P. ROSSI 1966 *Why families move*. Glencoe: The Free Press. Rossi found specific housing problems to be the most significant factor in the desire of a family to move.

20. Op. cit. *Nova.*
21. Op. cit. Gans, p. 149.
22. WHYTE, WILLIAM H. 1968 *The last landscape.* New York: Doubleday.
23. Op. cit. Gans, p. 145. He calls these 'definitional struggles, in which people "sorted themselves out" '.
24. MORRIS, R. and MOGEY, J. 1965 *The sociology of housing*, p. 104. London: Routledge and Kegan Paul. They point out that community-building alternates between friendship and friction.

Chapter 3

1. SIMMEL, G. *The sociology of Georg Simmel.* K. WOLFF (ed.), p. 409. Glencoe: The Free Press, 1950; London: Collier-Macmillan.
2. BOORSTEIN, D. 1963 *The decline of radicalism*, p. 22. New York: Random House. Boorstein attempts to link the production and consumption of products with community in a discussion of 'consumption communities'. These 'consist of people who have a feeling of shared well-being, shared risks, shared interests, and common concerns that come from consuming the same kinds of objects'.
3. Op. cit. Simmel. Part two. 'Quantitative aspects of the group.' Paul Goodman, a critic of American society, discusses the relation of community to numbers in the concept of 'right proportion'. The increase in numbers requires a greater proportion of life activities to take place in small groups under decentralized controls and with greater protection of civil liberties. P. GOODMAN 1960 *Growing up absurd.* New York: Random House.
4. WOLF, C. 1969 *Garrison community.* Westport, Connecticut: Greenwood. In the first chapter the author reviews the various approaches to the study of community and adopts Don Martindale's view that community is a complete social system: 'a total interhuman way of life'. In such a community, institutions are the collective solutions to basic problems. See also: D. MARTINDALE 1965 *Institutions, organizations and mass society.* Boston: Houghton Mifflin.
5. Op. cit. Wolf, p. 212.
6. Op. cit. Wolf, p. 259.
7. Op. cit. Park.
8. REYNOLDS, M. 1963 Little boxes. Reprinted in M. OKUM (ed.) 1970 *Great songs of the sixties*, pp. 158–160. Chicago: Quadrangle Books.
9. VIDICH, A., and BENSMAN, J. 1960 *Small town in mass society.* New York: Anchor Books.
10. Ibid. p. 320.
11. The debate over education in England, particularly regarding mass as opposed to elite education, was clearly stated in the eleven-plus controversy. The current discussion centres upon the expansion of higher

education. See: A. H. HALSEY, J. FLOUD, and C. A. ANDERSON 1961 *Education, economy and society: a reader in the sociology of education.* New York: The Free Press; London: Collier-Macmillan.

12. WILSON, B. Sects and society. In J. A. BANKS (ed.) *Studies in British society.* London: Thomas Crowell.
13. BELL, D. 1960 *The end of ideology*, p. 36. New York: The Free Press. London: Collier-Macmillan. See also: E. SHILS 1969 The theory of the mass society. In D. MINAR and S. GREER (eds.) *The concept of community.* Chicago: Aldine Publishing Company; London: Butterworth, 1970.
14. This can be stated in terms of systems theory as follows: a community is itself a system, but a community may also be regarded as part of a wider system. Another distinction is between society and community. The former has been defined as: '. . . a group of human beings sharing a self-sufficient system of action which is capable of existing longer than the life-span of an individual, the group being recruited at least in part by the sexual reproduction of members.' D. ABERLE, A. COHEN, A. DAVIS, M. LEVY, and F. SUTTON. 1967 The functional prerequisites of a society. In N. DEMERETH and R. PETERSON (eds.) *System, change and conflict.* New York: The Free Press. According to Wirth: 'Community has come to refer to group life from the standpoint of consensus' (op. cit. p. 166). He also writes: 'A community may be regarded as a state of existence whereas a society is a state of mind' (p. 328).
15. WHYTE, W. 1966. The outgoing life. In E. and M. JOSEPHSON (eds.) *Man alone*, p. 544. New York: Dell Publishing Company. There has been no agreement on a definition of group. One author terms a village a 'permanent group'. W. J. H. SPROTT 1958 *Human groups.* Harmondsworth: Penguin, p. 9. Bierstedt assumes that almost every small collective is a group and divides them as follows:

	consciousness of kind	*social interaction*	*social organization*
a. statistical	no	no	no
b. societal	yes	no	no
c. social	yes	yes	no
d. associational	yes	yes	yes

R. BIERSTEDT 1970 *The social order*, p. 281. New York: McGraw-Hill.

16. How long communities exist is not clear. D. Bonhoeffer calls the Christian community a 'brief single encounter: or a daily fellowship that lasts for years'. D. BONHOEFFER 1954 *Life Together.* J. W. DOBERSTEIN (trans.). London: SCM Press. There is the *intention* of continued association inherent in community that is usually not present in a group, but it is difficult to specify more than this.
17. SHERIF, M. and SHERIF, C. (eds.) 1964 *Reference groups.* New York: Harper and Row. This is a general discussion of reference group theory. One distinction is between studying groups as they affect individual behaviour and the study of individual behaviour within groups. Simmel is also relevant on this point. He writes: 'The groups with which the individual is affiliated constitute a system of coordinates, as it were, such

that each new group with which he becomes affiliated circumscribes him more exactly and more unambiguously. To belong to any one of these groups leaves the individual considerable leeway. But the larger the number of groups to which an individual belongs, the more improbable is it that other persons will exhibit the same combination of group affiliations, that these particular groups will intersect once again.' K. WOLFF and R. BENDIX (trans.) 1955 *Conflict and the web of group affiliations*, p. 140. New York: The Free Press.

18. FLOUD, J. Karl Mannheim. In T. RAISON (ed.) 1969 *The founding fathers of social science*, p. 212. Harmondsworth: Penguin.
19. Ibid. p. 213.
20. CAMERON, W. 1954. *Informal sociology*, p. 70. New York: Random House.
21. This is vividly illustrated by reference to a poem engraved at the Gestalt Institute, 12921 Euclid Avenue, Cleveland, Ohio and written by F. PERLS. It reads:

    I do my thing and you do your thing.
    I am not in this world to live up to your expectations.
    And you are not in this world to live up to mine.
    You are you and I am I
    And if by chance we find each other, it's beautiful.
    If not, it can't be helped.

    Unlike community, a group does not require concern for other members, or commitment to collective goals: the basis of structured commonality.

Chapter 4

1. Although this chapter attempts to discuss community in terms of identity in the religious sphere, it should be understood that these ideas are interrelated and are arbitrarily divided for purposes of illustration. The relation of religion to issues of personal identity has been succinctly noted by O'Dea as follows: '. . . individuals, by their acceptance of the values involved in religion and the beliefs about human nature and destiny associated with them, develop important aspects of their own self-understanding and self-definition.' T. O'DEA 1966 *The study of religion*, p. 15. Englewood Cliffs: Prentice-Hall. Religion provides an excellent example of the link between community and identity, and it is used as such here, rather than as a discussion of community and church, See also: Seminarians seek to experiment with communal living. *Christian Science Monitor* 22 December 1969.
2. MOORE, S. and MAGUIRE, K. 1970 *The dreamer not the dream*. London: Darton, Longman, and Todd. They argue that any assembly of people for worship, regardless of circumstances, 'cannot be representative of

that community of which the Christian celebration is properly the expression, for that community is man in all his depth and extent, his natural extendedness into his fellow humans and into the world that produces and feeds him' (p. 16). In their view, the church is a community that never meets.

3. Op. cit. Strauss, p. 3.
4. This is supported by theologians Moore and Maguire who flatly assert that what is happening in the church is a psychological transformation (op. cit. p. 5).
5. The term 'inauthentic' was originally used by Sartre to refer to man himself: 'Authenticity, it is almost needless to say, consists of having a true and lucid consciousness of the situation, in assuming the responsibilities and risks that it involves, in accepting it in pride or humiliation, sometimes in horror and hate.' SARTRE, J.-P. 1948 *Anti-semite and Jew.* G. BECKER (trans.) New York: Shocken Books. Etzioni applies the term to refer to a relationship, institution, or society 'if it provides the appearance of responsiveness while the underlying condition is alienating' (op. cit. p. 619).
6. SCHERER, J. 1966. Is the church a community? a case study. Unpublished paper. Syracuse University, East-African Centre, Syracuse, New York. This case is typical of Anglican parishes in many ways. See: D. MARTIN 1967 *The sociology of religion.* London: Heinemann.
7. BROTHERS, J. 1964 *Church and school.* Liverpool: Liverpool University Press.
8. WARD, C. Living in a new community. Unpublished paper presented to the Statistical and Social Inquiry Society for Ireland, 15 November 1968. See also: F. HOUTART, Sociologie de la paroisse comme assemblée eucharistique. *Social Compass* 1963 vol. 1, pp. 75–91. R. RHODES, Structure of the church's presence in the world today – through the church's own institutions. *Concilium,* 8–6 October 1970. The identification with locality is clear in the case of the local denominational church in Protestantism, even when the term 'parish' is not used. To understand the relationship with place in Judaism see: M. SKLARE, J. GREENBLUM, and B. RINGER 1969 *Not quite at home.* The American Jewish Committee: Institute of Human Relations.
9. Because religion is directed toward the inner life of individuals, its psychological manifestations are enormously important, but because these practices and beliefs are shared, they are also sociological in nature. Because of 'the complex interaction of personal experience and beliefs with social structure' the examination of religions will remain a critical area of investigation. J. BROTHERS 1971 *Religious institutions,* p. 90. London: Longmans.
10. COX, H. 1965 *The secular city.* New York: Macmillan. In the words of a journalist: 'The fatal flaw in man's past devotion to holiness has been his inability to sustain the illusion of the reality of sacred connections with strangers. Yet most of us are strangers to each other. As a result, we become mere objects or mysteriously evil or wholly invisible to each

other.' M. HELPER, Israel's incoherent response to an incoherent Arab world. *Saturday Review* 14 February 1970.

11. GREELEY, A. 1968 *The crucible of change*, p. 93. New York: Sheed and Ward. A useful overview of the relation of structure and religion is found in: B. SCHARF 1970 *The sociological study of religion.* London: Hutchinson.
12. Etzioni suggests that a major different between modern and traditional collectivism lies in their scope and pervasiveness and suggests that studying the difference in activation among various associations might be of value. It would appear a useful path to locate communal forms (op. cit. Chapter 16: The morphology of modern and post-modern societies, pp. 432–465).
13. There is a need for more imaginative approaches to the study of qualitative data. Survey techniques are often ineffective because members answer as they are expected to reply. See: J. SCHERER Qualitative data/trends: a methodological note. *Social Compass* Vol. XVIII, 1971/2.
14. FICHTER, J. 1967 The urban parish as a social group. J. BROTHERS (ed.) *Readings in the sociology of religion.* Oxford: Pergamon.
15. Ibid. p. 199.
16. BETTELHEIM, B. Obsolete youth. *Encounter* September 1969.
17. KENISTON, K. Youth, change and violence. *The American Scholar* Spring 1968, p. 228.
18. ERIKSON, E. 1963 Youth, fidelity and diversity. In E. ERICKSON (ed.) *The challenge of youth* (Originally published as *Youth: change and challenge*), p. 23. New York: Doubleday.

Chapter 5

1. SOP, N. *Encounter* November 1969.
2. JACKSON, B. 1969 *Working class community.* London: Routledge and Kegan Paul.
3. The term 'culture of poverty' is best described by O. LEWIS 1961 *The children of Sanchez.* New York: Random House. It refers to the self-perpetuating circle of poverty, ill health, lack of opportunity, and poor achievement. This concept has been critically attacked by J. ROACH and O. CUSSLIN: An evaluation of the concept 'culture of poverty'. *Social Forces* March 1967.
4. Op. cit. Jackson, p. 157. Working-class living-styles are similar to those described by Greeley in ethnic populations. According to Greeley, '. . . the ethnic collectively represents an attempt on the part of men to keep alive in their pilgrimage from peasant village to industrial metropolis, some of the diffuse, descriptive, particularistic modes of behaviour that were common in the past. The ethnic group was created only when the peasant communes broke up and was essentially an attempt to keep

some of the values, some of the informality, some of the support, some of the intimacy of the communal life in the midst of an impersonal, formalistic, rationalized, urban, industrialized society.' A. GREELEY, 1969 Why can't they be like us? Monograph. New York: Institute of Human Relations Press, No. 12, p. 18.

5. BERNSTEIN, B. A socio-linguistic approach to social learning. J. GOULD (ed.) 1965 In *Penguin survey of the social sciences.* Harmondsworth: Penguin.
6. DEUTSCHER, I. The social causes of social problems from suicide to delinquency. E. MIZRUCHI (ed.) 1967 *The substance of sociology.* New York: Meredith.
7. Problems of poverty in Great Britain have been described as 'a national disgrace.' See: Social reform in the centrifugal society. *New Society* 11 September 1969. The difficulties of dealing with these by traditional social-work methods are discussed by P. DANIEL Choosing the therapy. *New society* 17 July 1969, and in the United States in: I. DEUTSCHER and E. THOMPSON (eds.) 1968 *Among the poor.* New York, London: Basic Books.
8. TOWNSEND, P. and ABEL-SMITH, B. The meaning of poverty. *British Journal of Sociology* September 1962 provides an overall interpretation of the problem. See also: O. ORNATI 1966 *Poverty amid affluence.* New York: Twentieth Century Fund, or LARMER, J. and HOWE, I. 1969 *Poverty: views from the left.* New York: William Morrow.
9. This obvious statement has serious implications for political welfare programmes which have been, traditionally, based upon naïve views of the social consequences of poverty in terms of range, depth, and potency in developing personalities.
10. Harlem reflects the two factors of race and poverty which generally exist side by side in most U.S. cities. Blacks make up 42% of all families in metropolitan 'poverty areas' but only 6% of those families living in areas not classified as poor. H. SHEPPARD (ed.) 1970 *Poverty and wealth.* Chicago: Quadrangle. A study of boundaries within urban territories has been made in SUTTLES, G. 1968 *The social order of the slum.* Chicago, London: University of Chicago Press. According to Suttles, the moral order of the slum was based upon personalistic relationships with members of ethnic groups inside the group, and segmentation from the wider society permitting provincialism to dominate all life activities.
11. LOCKE, A. *Survey graphic* March 1925.
12. VERNEY, S. 1969 *People and cities*, p. 89. London: Collins.
13. FREID, M. and LEVIN, J. Some social functions of a slum. In B. FRIEDEN and R. MORRIS (eds.) 1968 *Urban planning and social policy.* New York, London: Basic Books. See also: J. BEKER and J. GELMAN The rural life of the urban poor (ibid.)
14. CLARKE, J. The early years of Adam Powell. In J. CLARKE (ed.) 1969 *Harlem, a community in transition*, p. 233. New York: Citadel Press. See also: F. FRAZIER 1964 *The Negro church in America.* Liverpool: Liverpool University Press.

15. Because soul embraces so many concepts, serving as an 'umbrella' under which many ideas congregate, it is difficult to define. It generally suggests the essence of blackness, based upon sincerity, intensity, and the commonality of the experience of black identity.
16. Op. cit. Jackson. He argues that working-class experience in essence 'feels the same' in spite of many changes (p. 166).
17. Op. cit. Clarke. K. CLARKE, interviewer. A conversation with James Baldwin (p. 130).
18. For a discussion of these changes see: F. COX, J. ERLICH, J. ROTHMAN, and J. TROPMAN (eds.) 1970 *Strategies of community organization.* Itasca, Illinois: F. E. Peacock. An anthropological statement of the changed approach to community development is found in W. GOODENOUGH 1966 *Cooperation in change.* New York: Russell Sage Foundation.
19. NEUWIRTH, G. A Weberian outline of a theory of community. Its application to the dark ghetto. *British Journal of Sociology* June 1969.

Chapter 6

1. LASSWELL, H. 1958 *Who gets what, when, how?* Cleveland, Ohio: The World Publishing Company.
2. O'BRIEN, A. Atheist in a foxhole *New Statesman* 3 January 1969.
3. EARISMAN, D. 1968 *Hippies in our midst: the rebellion beyond rebellion.* Philadelphia: The Fortress Press. Earisman makes this comparison on many points.
4. Op. cit. Greeley *The crucible of change* (p. 55).
5. SCHERER, J. Alternatives to halls. In J. BROTHERS and S. HATCH (eds.) 1971 *Residence and Student Life.* London: Tavistock.
6. A similar process occurs in many commune groups developing throughout the world. Examples of 'intentional communities' which try to structure spontaneity are numerous. See: *Directory of communes* listing projects, 'tribes, crashpads, and related phenomena in Great Britain and Europe'. The Commune Movement, BIT 141, Westbourne Park Rd. London W 11.
7. Op. cit. Simmel, p. 33.
8. K. KENISTON The transvaluation of utopia. In H. RUITENBECK (ed.) 1963 *Varieties of social theory.* New York: Dutton.
9. Simmel writes: 'If we did not have the power and right to rebel against tyranny, arbitrariness, moodiness, tactlessness, we could not bear to have any relation to people from whose characters we suffer . . . Our opposition makes us feel that we are not completely victims of circumstances' (op. cit. p. 19).
10. COSER, L. 1956 *The functions of social conflict.* Glencoe: The Free Press.

11. COLEMAN, J. 1957 *Community conflict.* Glencoe: The Free Press.

12. HOFSTADTER, R. Commencement address, 1968. *Columbia College Today* Spring 1968. The most eloquent statement of this was made by Cardinal Newman, who wrote: 'If I had to choose between a so-called university which dispenses with residence and tutorial superintendence and gave its degree to any person who passed an examination in a wide range of subjects and a university which had no professors or examinations at all, but merely brought a number of young men together for three or four years . . . If I were asked which of these two methods was the better discipline of the intellect . . . was the more successful in training, moulding, enlarging the mind, which sent men out more fitted for their secular duties, which produced better public men, men of the world, men whose names would descend to posterity, I have no hesitation in giving the preference to the latter.' *The idea of a university*, Discourse VI, Section 9. New York: Doubleday Image, 1959.

13. WILSON, L. Disjunctive processes in an academic milieu. In E. TIRYAKIAN (ed.) *Sociological theory, values and sociocultural change.* New York: Harper Torchbooks, 1963. London: Collier-Macmillan. D. Jenkins has summarized the advantages and disadvantages of the academic community as follows: the positive – helps to promote the pursuit of knowledge, leads to humility, patience, self-criticism and mutual dependence; the negative – triviality, lack of proportion, indecisiveness, and self-righteousness. See: D. JENKINS 1964 *The educated society.* London: Faber and Faber.

14. KERR, C. *The Daily Californian* 11 May 1967 Quoted by E. SAMPSON Two revolutions. In E. SAMPSON and H. KORN and associates (eds.) *Student activism and protest.* San Francisco: Jossey-Bass, 1970. See also: J. MILLET 1962 *The academic community.* New York, London: McGraw-Hill.

15. Op. cit. Etzioni, p. 642.

16. SCHERMERHORN, R. 1962 *Society and power.* New York: Oxford University Press.

17. NISBET, R. 1962 *Community and power.* New York: Oxford University Press.

18. SCHNEIDER, R. 1968 *Destiny of change*, p. 107. New York: Holt, Rinehart and Winston.

19. DURKHEIM, E. *The division of labor in society.* New York: The Free Press, 1933. Reprinted 1966. Preface to revised edition, p. 28.

20. HUGHES, E. 1943 *French Canada in transition* Chicago, London: University of Chicago Press, p. 3. In view of recent events in French Canada, many of Hughes's observations appear timely.

21. Ibid. p. 72.

22. Ibid. p. 44.

23. Ibid. p. 73.

24. Ibid. p. 211.

25. Ibid. p. ix.

Chapter 7

1. Op. cit. Bennis and Slater, p. 21.
2. FIRTH, R., HUBERT, J. and FORGE, A. 1970 *Families and their relatives*. London: Routledge and Kegan Paul. See also: D. SCHNEIDER and G. HOMANS, Kinship terminology and the American kinship system. *American Anthropologist* December 1955, pp. 1194–1208.
3. The term 'family' can be used to cover any set of relationships recognized by the participants. In analysis, the general concentration is upon the study of the functions which the unit performs in society. See: N. BELL and E. VOGEL Toward a framework for functional analysis of family behavior. In N. BELL and E. VOGEL (eds.) 1968 *A modern introduction to the family* Revised edition. New York: The Free Press; London: Collier-Macmillan.
4. The recent revision of Dr Spock's classic on child-rearing is an example of the distortion found in the use of this term. Spock was considered the 'father' of permissiveness because he advocated a more relaxed approach to child-care during the era of rigid scheduling, strict control, and regulated feeding. In his recent revision, he argues for more regulation and parental direction. Dr Spock thinks again. *Observer Magazine* January 1969.
5. LAING, R. D. 1967 *The politics of experience* p. 43. Harmondsworth: Penguin; New York: Pantheon, Laing has been the most articulate critic of the tyranny of family life, particularly the cruelties which accompany socialization of the child. See: LAING, R. D. and ESTERSON, A. 1964 *Sanity, madness, and the family*. London: Tavistock. A sceptical note regarding the influence of parental values upon children is found in: F. FURSTENBERG The transmission of mobility orientation in the family. *Social Forces* vol. 49, 4 June 1971, p. 595.
6. There has developed an extensive literature concerning child-rearing in the kibbutz. Some of the most popular are: SPIRO, M. 1958 *Children of the kibbutz*. Cambridge: Harvard University Press. RABIN, A. 1965 *Growing up in the kibbutz*. New York: Springer. BETTELHEIM, B. 1969 *The children of the dream*. New York: The Macmillan Company; London: Collier-Macmillan.
7. Bettelheim writes: 'In a pluralistic society such as ours, most of all in our urban centres, even the very young child is exposed to many different ways of solving life's problems. If nothing else, variations in our standards of living practically force him, from the earliest age, to question his family's way of life and to wonder for which way he will opt . . . Things are different in the kibbutz. There is little chance for any difference of opinion to crop up in the peer group because where would the ideas come from? It more or less takes an outside influence to raise the issues they might differ about' (op. cit. p. 219).
8. Spiro argues: 'In the absence of a specific social group – the family – to whom society delegates the function of socialization, reproduction etc., it has become necessary for the entire society to become a large extended

family. But only in a society whose members perceive each other psychologically as kin can it function as a family. And there would seem to be a population limit beyond which point individuals can no longer be perceived as kin. That point is probably reached when the interaction of its members is no longer face-to-face; in short, when it ceases to be a primary group. It would' seem probable, therefore, that only in a "familial" society, such as the kibbutz, is it possible to dispense with the family.' M. SPIRO, Is the family universal? In H. ROSS (ed.) *Perspectives on the social order*. New York: McGraw-Hill, 1963.

9. MILLER, D., SWANSON, G. 1958 *The changing American parent*. New York: John Wiley. The transformation of traditional sex roles is a most significant factor in changing patterns of child care.
10. Bloodworth states: 'The family came first, the individual second, much as among the best of the West the nation came first and the individual second. As for the country, this ran a poor third with the Chinese.' D. BLOODWORTH 1966 *The Chinese looking glass*. p. 101. New York: Farrar Straus and Gerous. On the other hand, it is dangerous to picture Chinese society as totally structured around the family. Latourette points out that 'Chinese society was an interplay of groups, some of them united by blood, some by economic ties, and some by political, professional or religious interests.' K. LATOURETTE 1967 *The Chinese – their history and culture*, p. 578. 4th revised edition. New York: Macmillan. See also: P. HO An historian's view of the Chinese family system. In M. BARASH and A. SCOURBY (eds.) *Marriage and the family*. New York: Random House, 1970.
11. ETZIONI, A. 1961 *A comparative analysis of complex organizations*. New York: The Free Press.
12. TOCH, H. 1965 *The social psychology of social movements*. London: Methuen; Indianapolis: Bobbs-Merrill. An attempt to measure values has been made by R. WARREN: Toward a non-Utopian normative model of the community. Paper read at American Sociological Association Meeting, San Francisco, September 1969.
13. KANTER, R. Commitment and social organization: a study of commitment mechanism in Utopian communities. *American Sociological Review* vol. 3, August 1968.
14. GERLACH, L. and HINE, V. 1970 *People, power change movements of social transformation*. Indianapolis: New York: Bobbs-Merrill.
15. REISS, A. The sociological study of communities. In R. WARREN (ed.) 1966 *Perspectives on the American community*. Chicago: Rand McNally.
16. SUSSMAN, M. The isolated nuclear family; fact or fiction. *Social Forces* Spring 1959.
17. Op. cit. Bennis and Slater.
18. MEAD, M. Youth revolt: the future is now. *Saturday Review* 10 January 1970. See also: M. MEAD 1970 *Culture and commitment*. New York: Doubleday. In this, Mead argues that the central problem of today is not identity but commitment: 'To what past, present or future can the idealistic young commit themselves?'

Chapter 8

1. NISBET, R. 1970 *The social bond*, p. 45. New York: Alfred Knopf. For an interesting discussion of bonding in all systems see: BERRIEN, K. 1968 *General and social systems*. New Brunswick: Rutgers University Press. According to Berrien, there are two kinds of chemical bonds: covalent (electrons are charged by two atoms) and ionic (ions of different charges held together by their actual attraction). Usually bonds are mixed and an optimum stable distance between molecules is characteristic of the atoms composing them. Using these concepts, Berrien suggests ways in which these ideas can be applied to social systems.
2. Science has always had a set of antithetical systems or attitudes; reductionist and holistic; or in Durkheimian terms, mechanistic and organic. The tension between objective measurement or an attempt to remove any personal qualities which interfere with reasoning and subjective insight (e.g. intuition, dreams), is also familiar. In terms of community, the distinction between community and society or association reflects this kind of differentiation.
3. TIGER, L. 1969 *Men in groups*, p. 21. London: Nelson. Tiger stresses the biological bonding propensity of all humans as a dependant variable in association. He argues that this leads to dominance in social roles, and consequently, aggression. The use of social bonding as an explanation for phenomena does not begin to suggest the close connection between social, cultural, and biological factors. It is not a convincing explanation for the complexity of social bonds found in community.
4. ADAMS, B. Interaction theory and social networks. *Sociometry* vol. XXX, 1, March 1967.
5. MACKENZIE, W. J. M. 1967 *Politics and social science*, p. 244. Harmondsworth: Penguin.
6. SILVERMAN, D. 1970 *The theory of organizations*. London: Heinemann. In this overview of organizational theory, Silverman argues that 'the nature of the social order that sociologists study and of the major characteristics of social reality thereby implied' is the fundamental issue of adopting different approaches to understanding organizations (p. 5). In Chapter 6, The action frame of reference, he succinctly summarizes the arguments for alternatives to the functionalist perspective which has dominated the study of organizations in recent years. His use of the word 'attachment' to describe membership in an organization provides a useful term to suggest the instrumental ties of person to organization without closing off the concept from the addition of more subjective or affective ties.
7. TURNER, V. 1969 *The ritual process: structure and anti-structure*, p. 96. London: Routledge and Kegan Paul.
8. WHYTE, W. 1956 *The organization man*. New York: Simon and Schuster; Harmondsworth: Penguin. According to Max Weber, 'Every social relationship which goes beyond the pursuit of immediately obtainable ends involves a relative degree of permanency between the same persons

and such relations cannot be limited to activities of a purely technical nature . . . Conversely, it is possible for a social relationship of primarily communal character, to manifest a type of behaviour on the part of its members, which is, either wholly or in part, motivated by considerations of expedience.' H. B. SECHER (translator) 1962 *Basic concepts in sociology: Max Weber*, p. 92. London: Peter Owen.

9. SLOTE, A. 1969 *Termination: the closing at Baker Plant.* New York: Bobbs Merrill.
10. ARENSBERG, C. and KIMBALL, S. 1965 *Culture and community*, p. 16. New York: Harcourt Brace and World.
11. BURNS, T. and STALKER, G. M. 1966 *The management of innovation*, p. 97. London: Tavistock. This study began as an attempt to understand an industrial concern as a 'community of people at work'.
12. KATZ, D. and KAHN, R. 1966 *The social psychology of organizations*, p. 222. New York: John Wiley and Sons.
13. The development of a new consciousness, particularly among the young, is a popular theme in current literature. The Bergers suggest, however, that the revolt against technology and the emerging countercultures will not negate the existence of a technological society and those who develop the skills to operate technology will become the power elite. Children of the lower-middle and working classes, who have been relatively unaffected by the upper-middle-class revolt against technology, will take over leadership by default, thereby strengthening, not weakening, the class system. P. BERGER and B. BERGER The blueing of America. *The New Republic* 3 April 1971.
14. TRILLING, L. Authenticity and the modern unconscious. *Commentary*, p. 39, September 1971.
15. DELESPESSE, M. 1966 *The church community – leaven and life style*, p. 4. Ottawa, Canada: The Catholic Centre of St. Paul University. Translated K. Russell.
16. Op. cit. Gerlach and Hine, p. 55.
17. Op. cit. Nisbet, *The social bond*, p. 81.
18. GREELEY, A. 1970 *The friendship game*, pp. 24–25. N.Y.: Doubleday.
19. BRUYN, S. T. H. 1966 *The human perspective in sociology: the methodology of participant observation.* Englewood Cliffs: Prentice-Hall. Bruyn defines social sciences in a wide perspective, arguing that empiricism must have a broader, more complex meaning than that used in the physical sciences. Although the argument for dealing with such issues has been almost a constant theme in social research, it must be restated again because it is so bitterly rejected by rigid empiricists, who would abandon the study of such problems until our methodological sophistication increased. Unfortunately, the importance of such problems grows and cannot await the development of adequate skills.
20. Since community studies have long been identified with functionalism, it is important to repeat that it is used in this discussion as an open system. M. WAX Myth and interrelationship in social science: illustrated through anthropology and sociology. In M. SHERIF and C. SHERIF (eds.) *Inter-*

disciplinary relationships in the social sciences. Chicago: Aldine Publishing Company, 1966. writes: 'From their inception, the studies of the exotic little community have been contributory to the development of a simply and powerful theoretical system – functionalism, in which the exotic community was treated as an isolated system balanced in dynamic equilibrium (homeostasis). To regard a Trobriand village as an isolated whole might be considered a minor error; to do the same for a New England city was an error of far greater magnitude.'

21. LABARRE, W. 1970 *The ghost dance*, p. 21. New York: Doubleday.

Chapter 9

1. ALLPORT, F. 1933 *Institutional behavior*, p. 510. Chapel Hill, North Carolina: University of North Carolina Press. Reprinted in: LYND, R. 1939 *Knowledge for what?* p. 188. New York: Grove Press.
2. Op. cit. Mackenzie, pp. 194–195.
3. Progressive educators saw the school as an attempt to deal with many facets of the child's life (the 'whole' child) and were willing to work towards a school community, but this conflicted with the professional image of teachers as educational specialists, The result is that the morality of the institution may be far afield from that of the community. For example, a mythical teacher may be able to escape the implications of his institutional behaviour in grading examinations within the educational context, but must face the consequences in a community which might be striving to eliminate inequality via selection.
4. The increase in numbers and range of association has become so marked in advanced technological societies that it is possible to conceive of a multiplicity of memberships as a form of wider societal integration similar to Durkheim's view of the division of labour. As we adopt many different associational ties, which cover an ever wider geographical, personal, professional, and social area, loyalties are wider, and co-ordination between various groupings is an imperative. See: J. PENNOCK and J. CHAPMAN 1969 *Voluntary associations.* New York: Atherton.
5. Op. cit. Schneider, p. 8.
6. GOFFMAN, E. 1961. On the characteristics of total institutions. *Asylums.* Garden City, New York: Anchor Books; Harmondsworth: Penguin.
7. ILLICH, I. 1970 *Deschooling society*, p. 1. New York, London: Harper and Row. London: Calder and Boyars, 1971.
8. Ibid. p. 55.
9. FRANKENBERG, R. 1966 *Communities in Britain*, pp. 241–242. Harmondsworth: Penguin Books.
10. SHANKS, M. A farewell to the sixties. *The Times* (London) 14 November 1969. He writes: 'Whereas in the sities we have all been trying, in the interests of economic competitiveness, to hurry forward the process of

change, in the seventies the debate will be how we can live with and master our Frankenstein monster.'

11. SCHON, D. 1971 *Beyond the stable state*. London: Temple Smith. Schon views belief in the stable state as the way in which we protect ourselves from threats inherent in change, although, in fact, no institution is stable and all are actively threatened.
12. GOFFMAN, E. 1961 *Encounters*. Indianapolis, Ind.: Bobbs-Merrill. Goffman writes: 'This "effectively" expressed pointed separateness between the individual and his putative role I shall call role distance. A short-hand is involved here: the individual is actually denying not the role but the virtual self that is implied in the role for all accepting performers' (p. 108).
13. GOODE, W. J. 1966 A theory of role strain. In W. J. GOODE (ed.) *The dynamics of modern society*. New York: Atherton.
14. LAPPING, A. Community careless. *New Society*, 9 April 1970. The Peckham Experiment in the late twenties and the thirties was an attempt to develop family health centres. Led by Dr Scott Williamson, a health centre was established to meet the needs of all ages. It has been described by J. COMERFORD 1947 *Health the unknown – the story of the Peckham experiment*. London: Hamish Hamilton.
15. PASSMORE, J. Paradise now. *Encounter* November 1970, p. 9.
16. Op. cit. Goode.
17. SYRETT H. Challenges facing urban universities. *School and society* February 1970.
18. Op. cit. Goffman, p. 3.
19. Op. cit. Cox, Erlich, Rothman, and Tropman. In terms of research, it means the greater use of longitudinal studies, more effective interviewing and observing, multivariate analysis, and other sophisticated skills in conducting community studies.
20. Op. cit. Arensberg and Kimball, p. 33.

Chapter 10

1. DEWEY, J. 1929 *The public and its problems*, p. 154. New York: Holt and Sons.
2. DEUTSCH, K. 1966 *The nerves of government*. New York: The Free Press; London: Collier-Macmillan.
3. ARANGUREN, J. 1967 *Human communication*. London: Weidenfeld and Nicolson, p. 12.
4. MILLS, C. W. 1958 *The power elite*. New York: Oxford University Press. A reply to Mills can be found in: D. MCQUALL 1968 *Towards a sociology of mass communications*. London: Collier-Macmillan. For a practical guide on ways viewers could influence mass media, see: N. JOHNSON 1967 *How to talk back to your television set*. New York: Atlantic-Little Brown.

5. SCHRAG, P. No place to grow. *Saturday Review* 21 March 1970.
6. Op. cit. Dewey, p. 5.
7. BOTT, E. 1957 *Family and social network.* London: Tavistock, p. 216.
8. BOTT, E. 1971 *Family and social network.* Second edition. London: Tavistock; New York: The Free Press of Glencoe, 1972. In the chapter entitled 'Reconsiderations', p. 249.
9. MITCHELL, J. CLYDE 1969 The concept and use of social networks. In J. C. MITCHELL (ed.): *Social networks in urban situations.* Manchester: Manchester University Press.
10. Op. cit. Bott, 1971, Reconsiderations, p. 304.
11. Op. cit. Scherer. In Brothers and Hatch (eds.) *Residence and student life.*
12. Op. cit. Mitchell. The difficulties facing the researcher in studying social networks are formidable, since the structure of the network can change with ease and speed. To locate all the links in any one person's network requires intensive study, and any given follow-up might include a wide social area through any given period of time.
13. Ibid. Mitchell points out that network analysis complements institutional analysis. In the bibliography included in this book, one can see that, in spite of its recent history, network analysis has become increasingly popular among researchers in a variety of social settings.
14. Several interesting attempts to develop chains of familiarity between persons in given localities have suggested that there are ways to measure and evaluate the range of contacts in very wide networks.

Chapter 11

1. Op. cit. Moore and Maguire, p. 131.
2. This is the structural–functional approach. Our approach has been to begin with the actors or participants and then look for the structures, noting that human interaction is always structured. For a definition of structure, I have adopted Redfield's: 'All social structure is not only a system of relationships of existing kinds of ties between people and doings done by kinds of people, but also a system of norms and expectancies.' R. REDFIELD 1955 *Little community.* Chicago: University of Chicago Press, p. 46.
3. COOLEY, C. 1902 *Human nature and the social order.* New York: Scribners. See also B. MOTT 1969 *Supergrow.* New York: Dutton
4. Strong criticism of theory without empirical referents is found consistently in the writing of C. Wright Mills, Robert Merton, and others in the decade 1950–1960.
5. Op. cit. Greeley, *The crucible of change*, p. 78. Another view is that of Keniston who writes: 'We need a more generous tolerance for synthetic and constructive formulations. Instead of concentrating on the

possible bad motives from which they arise (the genetic fallacy) or on the possible bad consequences which might ensue from their interpretation (the progenitive fallacy), we must learn to assess them in terms of their present relevance, depth and approriateness' (op. cit. p. 114, in *Varieties of modern social theories*).

Irving Howe goes further when he states that criticisms have been muted in the last few years because sociology itself has become institutionalized. 'During the greater part of the bourgeois era, intellectuals preferred alienation from the community to alienation from themselves. Precisely this choice made possible their boldness and strength, precisely this lack of roots gave them speculative power.' New styles of leftism. In I. HOWE (ed.) *The radical anthology*, p. 73. New York: The American Library.

6. DOUGLAS, M. 1970 *Natural symbols*, p. 1. London: Barrie and Rockliff; New York: Pantheon.

Postscript

1. FARSON, R. How could anything that feels so bad be so good? *Saturday Review* 6 September 1969.
2. Robert Boguslaw writes that 'a new breed of Utopians' or systems designers are in control of complex systems. This is brought about 'by the more or less deliberate exclusion of the most significant variables from the design process'. Choices become matters of priority, goals and values are translated into alternative programmes and significantly, these translated options eliminate many subtle distinctions and variations between ends and means. R. BOGUSLAW 1965 *The new Utopians: a study of system design and social change*. Englewood Cliffs, New Jersey: Prentice-Hall.
3. Op. cit. Minar and Greer, p. 9.
4. KRAFT, J. 1966 *Profiles in power*, p 13.. New York: The New American Library.

Index